A PLUME BOOK

HOW TO EXERCISE WHEN YOU'RE EXPECTING

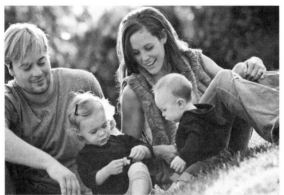

John Gaughan

LINDSAY BRIN, C.P.T. AND B.S.E. Exercise Science, is a fitness and nutrition expert and a former NFL cheerleader. For nearly fifteen years, she's been helping women achieve healthier bodies and minds. She has starred in, choreographed, and designed thirteen fitness DVDs just for moms. Her most recent ventures include not only becoming an author, but an infomercial and network TV.

Brin's lifelong passion for fitness developed while growing up and watching her mother teach aerobics. Since then she has become a fitness expert for magazines such as *Fit Pregnancy* and *Mom & Baby* and a contributor to online sites specializing in pre- and postnatal health. Leading research facilities use Brin's DVDs to certify fitness professionals. She is also a spokesperson for Fertility Lifelines, helping women become mothers.

Brin is an approachable, real, and inspiring resource for moms of all ages. Her faith and the strength of her family have helped her get where she is today. She lives in the suburbs of St. Louis with her husband, David, their little girl, and their baby boy.

To find out more about who Lindsay Brin is, and not just what she does, please visit her blog, lindsaybrin.com. You'll also see the good, the bad, and the ugly pictures of her getting her body back, with week-by-week photos starting from the day she got home from the hospital with her daughter and her son.

She'd love to hear from you! Chat with her on Facebook, Twitter, or her blog.
facebook.com/momsintofitness
twitter.com/lindsaybrin

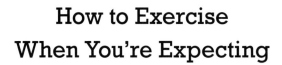

How to Exercise
When You're Expecting

Also by Lindsay Brin

The Cheerleader Fitness Plan

How to
EXERCISE
When You're
EXPECTING

For the **9 MONTHS** of Pregnancy
and the **5 MONTHS** It Takes
to Get Your Best Body Back

LINDSAY BRIN, C.P.T., B.S.E.

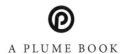

A PLUME BOOK

PLUME
Published by Penguin Group

Penguin Group (USA) Inc., 375 Hudson Street, New York, New York 10014, U.S.A. • Penguin Group
(Canada), 90 Eglinton Avenue East, Suite 700, Toronto, Ontario, Canada M4P 2Y3 (a division of Pearson
Penguin Canada Inc.) • Penguin Books Ltd., 80 Strand, London WC2R 0RL, England • Penguin Ireland,
25 St. Stephen's Green, Dublin 2, Ireland (a division of Penguin Books Ltd.) • Penguin Group (Australia),
250 Camberwell Road, Camberwell, Victoria 3124, Australia (a division of Pearson Australia Group
Pty. Ltd.) • Penguin Books India Pvt. Ltd., 11 Community Centre, Panchsheel Park, New Delhi – 110 017,
India • Penguin Books (NZ), 67 Apollo Drive, Rosedale, North Shore 0632, New Zealand (a division
of Pearson New Zealand Ltd.) • Penguin Books (South Africa) (Pty.) Ltd., 24 Sturdee Avenue, Rosebank,
Johannesburg 2196, South Africa

Penguin Books Ltd., Registered Offices: 80 Strand, London WC2R 0RL, England

First published by Plume, a member of Penguin Group (USA) Inc.

First Printing, April 2011
7   9   10   8   6
Copyright © Moms Into Fitness, Inc., 2011
Illustrations by Kevin Swift Art

Ⓟ REGISTERED TRADEMARK—MARCA REGISTRADA

LIBRARY OF CONGRESS CATALOGING-IN-PUBLICATION DATA

Brin, Lindsay.
    How to exercise when you're expecting : for the 9 months of pregnancy and the 5 months it takes to get
your best body back / Lindsay Brin.
        p.   cm.
    Summary: "From the author of "The Cheerleading Fitnees Book" is this new book on how to exercise
during pregnancy. With workout descriptions and illustrations to help expectant mothers stay fit during the nine months of pregnancy, and how to get back into shape after the baby is born"—Provided by
publisher.
    Includes bibliographical references.
    ISBN 978-0-452-29685-5 (pbk.)
    1. Physical fitness for pregnant women.   2. Exercise for pregnant women.   I. Title.
    RG558.7.B75 2011
    618.2'44—dc22
                                                                                    2010050221

Printed in the United States of America
Set in Minion Pro and Rockwell
Designed by Victoria Hartman

PUBLISHER'S NOTE

Every effort has been made to ensure that the information contained in this book is complete and accurate. However, neither the publisher nor the author is engaged in rendering professional advice or services to the individual reader. The ideas, procedures, and suggestions contained in this book are not
intended as a substitute for consulting with your physician. All matters regarding your health require
medical supervision. Neither the author nor the publisher shall be liable or responsible for any loss or
damage allegedly arising from any information or suggestion in this book.

While the author has made every effort to provide accurate telephone numbers and Internet addresses
at the time of publication, neither the publisher nor the author assumes any responsibility for errors, or
for changes that occur after publication. Further, the publisher does not have any control over and does
not assume any responsibility for author or third-party Web sites or their content.

BOOKS ARE AVAILABLE AT QUANTITY DISCOUNTS WHEN USED TO PROMOTE PRODUCTS OR SERVICES. FOR
INFORMATION PLEASE WRITE TO PREMIUM MARKETING DIVISION, PENGUIN GROUP (USA) INC., 375 HUDSON
STREET, NEW YORK, NEW YORK 10014.

For Nelly, Bubby, and Honey

CONTENTS

Part II : Post-Pregnancy

Part III : Lifestyle

ACKNOWLEDGMENTS

So many people dedicated their time to get this book published! It's hard to know where to begin, so here goes.

To my editor, Cherise, I wish I could go inside your brain and pick out some of the knowledge in there! Your intelligence is unreal. And it was a pleasure working with you through the birth of your two lil' ladies.

Kate, I don't know how you do it. But thank you for always staying on top of me and making sure things got done.

Scott, thank you for finding me an outlet to say everything I have to say! Who knew being an author would have been in my future? I owe that to you.

Gary, your writing amazes me. And I couldn't be happier. For the lump of unorganized data and exercises being made into this book—wow!

Kevin, thank you for countless hours of staring at pictures of me and making illustrations out of them, all two hundred of them!

My family, from cheering me on and never doubting I could do it to watching the kids while I pulled all-nighters to get this done, I couldn't have done it without you. Some people just say that, but I really mean it.

Brent, thank you for supporting this whole business idea, knowing what to do, and helping me find my way.

Mom S., thanks for the hours you spent taking care of both Rylan and Taylor and for the encouragement you always gave me. Your support and confidence never wavered; thank you.

Dad S., thanks for your wonderful illustrations and editing skills. Next time we'll have to put your illustrations in the contract! Your humor and intelligence has been an incredible help not only in forming my business projects, but in molding me into the mom I want to be.

Dad, I've always been a daddy's girl! Your love and support has never stopped, and the confidence you have in me is what I hope to carry through. For all the time that you give to make it all happen, I love you.

Mom, it all began after Taylor was born. You'll never know how much I appreciate the time you took out of your own life to support this project, from the hours she spent in the Baby Björn to the hours you spent catering to me. I want to be just like you.

David, I'm still not sure how you put up with me sometimes! I really, truly know none of this would have happened without you. No matter what wacky idea I have, you are there to support it and be my number one fan. I'm not sure what more a wife could ask for. So thank you for not only supporting me and loving me, but for putting up with me!

Rylan and Taylor, I'm sorry for all the days I did not spend time with you. But writing this book and being a working mother makes me a better mother; I promise. I love you both.

INTRODUCTION

We often refer to a child's birth as a blessed event. There's a reason for that. For many women, having a child is the ultimate experience of their adult life. Sure, there's no more important duty your body will be asked to perform than to bear a child. But you are asked to put on anywhere from fifteen to thirty-five pounds within nine months. This would be hard for anyone to lose. But the good news is a majority of that weight will go when the baby is born. The rest is up to you and how you take care of yourself now . . . meaning don't gain too much too fast.

Whether you think of it as expressing her reproductive destiny, getting knocked up, an "oops," or as her fulfilling her maternal instinct to nurture and protect, having a baby is one of the defining moments of a woman's life. From the moment she hears the news from a doctor or sees the two red lines on a home pregnancy kit, her life is going to be changed forever. Or if you're like me you cried when your husband told you that you were pregnant after the nurse called with HCG numbers, and were shocked to be carrying twins. Some women are scared out of their minds and optimistic but pessimistic about how it's all going to turn out. I hope for you and your family it's a time of joy and optimism, but if it's not—you are not alone in being scared. I was Nervous Nelly, even knowing all I know about pregnancy.

Not only is your life going to change, but your body is going to undergo a series of changes—some wonderful, some wacky, some initially frightening—that could potentially leave you looking like a different person than you were before your pregnancy.

I think you either have it easy or you have it hard. You enjoy it or you don't. But either way the goal is to get to forty weeks. If you're like me the "glow" is green to gills, "tired" is insomnia instead, and "loving every minute of it" is "I am ready to jump out of my skin."

Let's face it, if you picked up this book, you did so because, as thrilled as you are about the life-changing events surrounding the birth of your child(ren), the one thing you want to see undone or to be able to go back to is your best pre-pregnancy body—or even better. Yes, it can be done, and you can look better than you did in high school! You want to be that "hot mom"! You know, the one everyone comments on: "You can't be serious! You just had a baby six months ago?" "Look at you! I thought you were the baby's nanny, not her mother!" Vain? Maybe, but I know I wanted to be *that* mom.

I also know that many of you are interested in staying fit during pregnancy. Whether it's because of your own personal experience or because you saw a friend or family member struggle with losing the weight gained during pregnancy, you want to do whatever you can to stay healthy and fit during your pregnancy. Or, like many of my good friends, you gained sixty pounds with your first child and realized how un-fun it was getting that weight off. Or you could still be carrying weight from the first one and don't want to be extra-overweight by the time this one pops out. Or you do it because you know you have to or it's your only way to de-stress with three other kids at home. Or you work out on occasion and have decided now is the time to really take care of yourself (like the 4 percent of women who are more active during pregnancy than non-pregnancy[1]), or the doctor said you have to! Either way, we just know that working out now will help you get your body back faster—studies show 40 percent faster.

Not only will you benefit from this emphasis on pre- and post-pregnancy fitness, but your newborn, your other children, and your partner will as well. Why? Having and raising a child takes an enormous amount of energy. (I'm not telling you moms anything you don't already know!) By being fit and feeling good about yourself and your body, you will have more of the energy and the enthusiasm that it takes to be a mom. No one wants to drag their feet throughout the day.

And when my husband dangles the running shoes, code for "Please leave and come back normal," I realize we all struggle with caretaking issues. What do I mean? Well, we women are by nature givers and providers. When we have kids, we have to sacrifice some of ourselves and our time and energy to devote to them. A lot of women feel guilty for doing anything for themselves. Let me tell you straight up from the start, the concept of the Supermom and the all-giving and no-receiving mom can lead to problems. I'm no psychologist, but I do know this: In order to better take care of others, you have to start by taking care of yourself! If you're not in good shape physically and mentally, you won't be as effective in carrying out your mothering responsibilities as you could be. So, that's Lindsay's Attitude **Rule #1: No Guilt.** Besides, with the program I've devised, you won't be spending hours and hours away from your family sweating in a gym or out on the road running miles and miles. You get it done in fifteen to fifty minutes and your kids can be by your side.

This book is based on cutting-edge information from top research facilities. I will guide you through a healthy pregnancy and crack down on losing the baby weight. It all starts with a healthy pregnancy and gaining only the recommended amount of weight, which is no more than twenty-five to thirty-five pounds if you're carrying one baby; the average woman gains 27.5 pounds.[2] Now, if you've already been through pregnancy and you gained more, do not fret. There is nothing you can do about the past; there is only something you can do for the future. You can use this book even if you had your baby five years ago—simply skip the pregnancy chapter.

Again, taking care of your family means taking care of yourself. Spending some time working out isn't selfish; it's smart.

Whom This Book Is Intended For

Even if you aren't pregnant and are just beginning to plan your family, this book can help you achieve the level of fitness and the goal weight to get you on the right path. I would love it if every woman got herself to her healthiest weight and fitness level before getting pregnant. I know that's not always the case, and to be honest, it isn't always necessary. However, if you think about getting your body back after childbirth, you'll understand why it is beneficial to be in the best shape possible pre-pregnancy. (Also, keep in mind I'm a pre- and postnatal fitness professional and I want everyone to feel the best about their body and their health! Having a healthy and positive body image leads to increased confidence and better health. It's confidence, not cockiness. Both play a large role in being a woman.)

If you are pregnant with a singleton or twins, as long as it's a healthy pregnancy and you have your doctor's permission you will benefit from every aspect of this book, from the non-worker-outer to the exercise vet, whether you've had no kids or eight kids. If you are pregnant with twins, you will have to take extra caution throughout your workout. Cardiovascular exercise is not recommended and you should stop exercising around twenty-two weeks. You can read more rules on page 7 of the exercise design. Just know you don't have to like working out, or eating tofu and broccoli—if you're all about getting it done in the least amount of time with the least amount of thought, this book is for you!

HOW TO GET YOUR BODY BACK INTO SHAPE AFTER BABY, WHETHER THIS IS YOUR FIRST BABY OR YOUR SEVENTH:

Rule #2: Do Not Gain More Than the Amount of Weight Your Doctor(s) Recommend! That's it in a sippy cup! The more you are able to stick to a nutrition and exercise program that helps you to control the amount of weight you gain during pregnancy, the easier it will be post-pregnancy to get your body back to where it was before pregnancy. If you don't, you're looking at more than five months to get that body back!

Obviously, then, the better shape you are in pre-pregnancy and the more accustomed you are to working out and not giving in to every cheeseburger craving, the better. Just as obvious, this book is intended for women who are already pregnant and want to begin a wellness program.

The American Congress of Obstetricians and Gynecologists' (ACOG) recent guidelines state that if you are not physically active before getting pregnant or if you have a medical condition you should talk with your doctor to plan a safe exercise program. So that means you should take this book with you and ask your doctor if it's OK for you to do the Beginner's Pregnancy Program. And you will probably want to stick to a maximum of twenty minutes of exercise three times a week through your first trimester.[3] If you don't have a history of exercising regularly, don't worry. This book will show you how you can do a program that will carry you through each of the trimesters and beyond.

Some of you have already gained sixty pounds from either this pregnancy or the previous one. Don't worry! This program will work for you too—but let's be honest, it might take you a little bit longer to lose that weight post-pregnancy. Your body is a fat-burning machine right after pregnancy, so we need to take advantage of that when we can!

And to my exercise vets: You will learn so much and find a good challenge within the workouts, although during pregnancy you will be the ones I will lecture for going too hard. When we exercise too hard, the blood flow goes to our muscles and not as much to our baby!

Finally, this book is also intended for women who have already given birth, whether it was five days or five years ago. I believe that it is both never too early and never too late to begin a fitness program.

Rule #3: No Excuses! What good does complaining about being in your thirties (or forties) and not being able to eat like you did in your twenties do? You can't lose weight by talking! And you simply cannot eat like you did in high school. I'm all about being straightforward and no bull crap, so leave your excuses at the door (or in your maternity closet)! It's time to work— but you don't have to dedicate an hour or two to working out, I promise! And you don't have to give up your favorite foods or the inevitable trip to the drive-through!

Rule #4: No Looking Back! For those of you who gave birth years ago and still haven't gotten the pregnancy weight off, this book is for you! And don't despair. You can't change the past, but you can change the future. Don't waste valuable time and energy kicking yourself for what you didn't do. Expend that energy kicking yourself into gear today!

I've structured the book so that if you aren't pregnant, you can skip Part I (which has a fitness plan for while you are pregnant) and go immediately to parts II and III—post-pregnancy and lifestyle plans.

So Here's the Skinny

A woman's body is made to bear a child. In order to do that, you will have to gain some weight. For most women that will ideally be somewhere between fifteen and thirty-five pounds. (See page 22 for the newest guidelines on recommended weight gain for singletons and twins.) You'll put that weight on in nine months' time. No matter how you look at it, that's a significant amount of weight to gain in that time frame. Losing that much weight would be hard for anyone. The good news is that the pregnancy weight will go between the time the baby is born and six weeks post-baby. The rest is up to you and how you take care of yourself. You're left with loose skin, loose muscles, and probably a few more pounds than going into the pregnancy.

You may be asking yourself where all of this weight comes from. A majority of it comes from the baby itself (seven to eight pounds) and your increasing muscle tissue and fluid (four to seven pounds). Other sources of weight gain are the placenta and amniotic fluid that protect the baby (three to four pounds), increased size of your breasts (approximately one pound) and uterus (two pounds), increased blood volume (three pounds), and finally increased body fat (five or more pounds).[4]

The average weight gain for pregnant women giving birth to a single child is 27.5 pounds. If you've already given birth and you gained more than that during your pregnancy, don't fret. We can still whip you into the kind of shape you want to be in. If you listen to your doctor and gain the recommended amount I guarantee that in five months you will have a stronger, leaner stomach than before.

If you've gained more than twenty-five or thirty pounds, following my program will allow you to get your body back within six to nine months, all depending on the amount you gained. That's right, in less than or equal to the amount of time it took you to put on that weight, you will lose it all and even more!

I know a lot of you are used to hearing claims about miraculous weight loss in weeks. Well, some women do experience those kinds of miracles by following those plans or taking those pills. As a health and fitness professional, I can tell you this: Those results aren't typical, and they may not be advisable. My program is a sane, sensible, and *safe* method for maintaining your health while losing weight.

My Journey to Motherhood

I have been in the situation you have all been in or are about to be in. Several years ago my husband and I started our quest to become parents. And after three years, we finally welcomed our first daughter, Taylor. We were especially grateful, since our journey to parenthood was such a difficult one. Like one in four Americans, we struggled with infertility issues. I was twenty-seven when we first learned that our only option was in vitro fertilization (IVF). What followed was a series of injections, tests, three IVFs, two losses (one being Taylor's twin), weight gain, and an emotional roller-coaster ride. Before actually undergoing each IVF cycle, I went through weeks of two to four daily injections. No fun!

But we did have to laugh and keep our sense of humor about it all. David, a practicing dentist, was skilled with the needle and with the verbal jab. He'd give me the costly injection and say, "Here's that Fendi purse you wanted," or "Here's those silk curtains for the dining room."

The injections messed with my hormones big-time, and my mood swings made the Wall Street ups and downs look like a flat line. I was told to monitor my weight carefully, since the hormone injections and steroids also did a number on my body. I was able to keep my trying-to-get-pregnant weight gain down to ten pounds. That means that my pre-baby weight gain was ten pounds and I wasn't even pregnant yet. I had friends who also went through the pre-IVF dance and wound up gaining sixty! But it was all worth it.

By my fourteenth week of pregnancy the scale showed I hadn't gained any weight, which my doctor said was OK because I had that ten-pound cushion from before. I had lost a few fat pounds as my metabolism sped up, and I'd gained a few baby pounds, so the scale showed a level weight. I wish I could say the fat pounds came off because of the way I was eating and working out, but it was from having my head in the toilet. I worked out, but ate whatever I could get down!

Now, this "eating whatever" changed during my second trimester after a five-pound weight gain in one week and an energy slump. At that point, every time I walked into my doctor's exam room and saw the scale, I could swear I saw it cringing at the sight of me! Well, back at ya, Ms. Scale. I was cringing at the sight of you. I know some of you hate looking at the scale, but it is a great tool in keeping you on track. Trust me, your doctor doesn't weigh you for embarrassment! If you hate it that much, just turn around on the scale and don't look; I'm sure your doctor will tell you if you're off track!

In the end, my weight gain leveled off, and I was a total of nineteen pounds heavier than I'd been before pregnancy. But I was twenty-nine pounds heavier than my usual weight. In the four months after Taylor was born I lost thirty-one pounds. (All nineteen pregnancy pounds were lost within the first ten weeks and once I stopped breast-feeding. Then I lost the additional ten pounds from before and a bonus two pounds!) I wish it had been easy and I could say it just fell off. But, like most moms out there, I had to work hard to get it off. I do know two moms for whom the weight just fell off without working at it, and if that's you—great, but let's concentrate on getting you strong and healthy.

Rule #5: If You Want Your Muscles to Bounce Back, You Have to Use Them. You can't run a marathon without a little training, right? So you can't expect your muscles to bounce back unless you do toning exercises. Pregnancy leaves you with loose muscles six weeks postpartum, and training them will pull them in like a corset.

And after my fourth IVF I was lucky enough to get pregnant again. I started off thinner this time around, as I literally walked off the set of my fitness

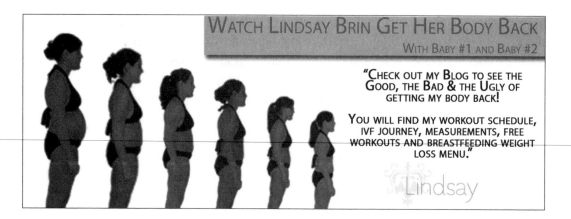

DVD filming and into the egg retrieval room. In the end I gained twenty-four pounds, spent a total of sixteen weeks on bed rest, and had to have my gall bladder removed. So I was left with lots of the jiggly, but a precious baby boy too! You can see the good, the bad, and the ugly on my blog, lindsaybrin.com. I posted all my pictures from pregnancy through one year postpartum, including the first day home after my C-section.

How to Use This Book

I've divided this book into three parts:

- The three trimesters of pregnancy, weeks four through forty
- The three phases of post-pregnancy, weeks zero to fourteen
- Ongoing weight maintenance, four to five months and beyond

In each of the three parts, you will find workouts specifically targeted to the phase of your life you are in. As you move through your pregnancy, exercises such as push-ups just aren't possible for you to do—unless you have really, really long arms! I modify each phase, keeping in mind the safety of your unborn child, your energy level, evolving physical changes, and the need to add variety to your routine. Maybe most important, I keep in mind how busy you are. My program doesn't require a significant investment of time or money.

As I stated earlier, if you have already given birth, no matter how long ago, you can skip to Part II of the book and follow the program outlined there. I'd love it if you read through the information in Part I so that if you are planning another addition to your family, you'll know what to expect as you move through each trimester.

I'm not only interested in seeing you get back your pre-pregnancy body (or getting back the body you had in high school or college); I want you to adopt an outlook and a routine that will help you maintain those results for the long term. We need to get rid of the easy-fix mentality. Just like stretch mark creams, there is no easy fix! Unfortunately, a cream cannot penetrate the skin enough to prevent stretch marks. Only growing at a steady rate and good genes can do that. But skin changes are normal, so do me a favor and use lotion for itchy skin, not to prevent cellulite and stretch marks. When somebody does invent one that works I will be the first one to eat my words and use it!

Pregnancy is one of the most eventful and life-changing periods in our lives. I know that at least eight hundred people told me that my life would never be the same after having a child. And it's true, so while we're at it, let's make other changes as well—working out regularly, eating more healthily, and more fully enjoying what your bodies are capable of!

PART I

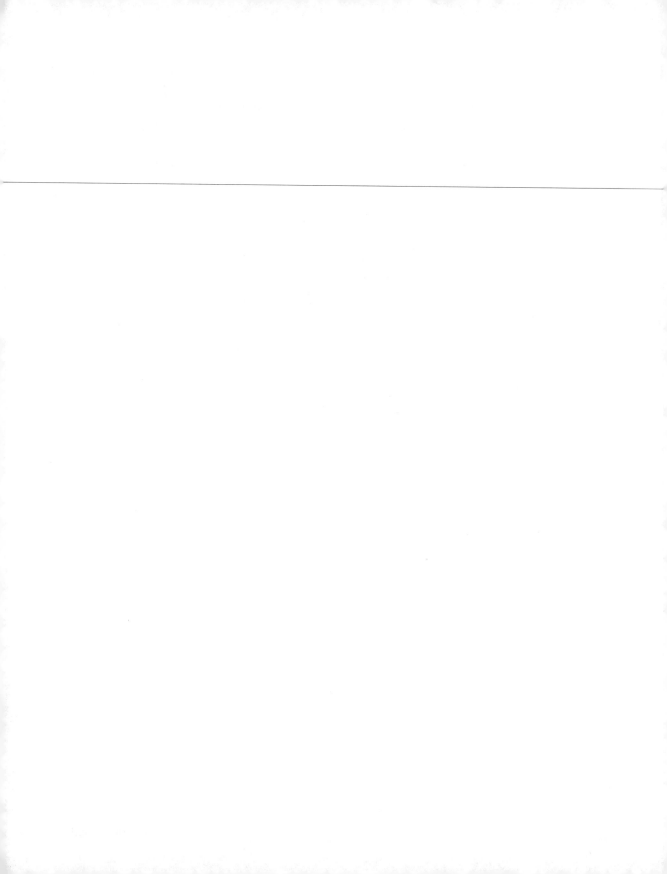

Pregnancy

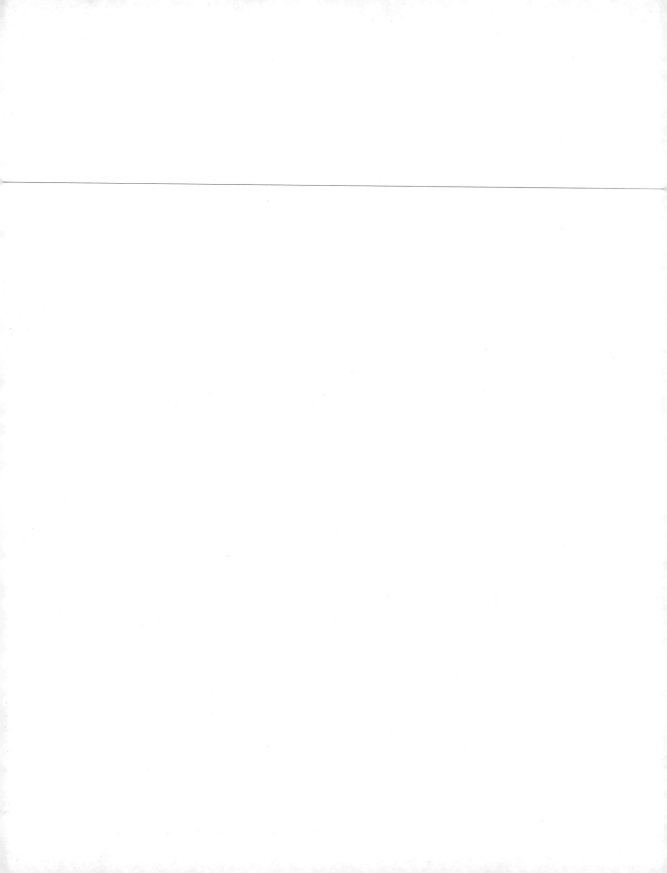

· 1 ·

WHAT TO EXPECT
WHEN YOU'RE EXERCISING

Before we get involved in anything, most of us women want and need some information. We typically don't plunge ahead into activities, relationships, jobs, or friendships without first—or at least shortly thereafter—getting the scoop from a friend, family member, coworker, or even a professional. As with buying a new crib, you do some digging, engage in some intelligence gathering. You want to know if the colors will match the old armoire, but more important, if it's safe!

I also have no doubt that when you got pregnant or were thinking of getting pregnant, you talked to friends, coworkers, and family, and consulted with some experts. There were lots of books, magazine articles, mothering wisdom, and other information presented to my husband and me, but that didn't prevent us from running to the emergency room when I spotted during pregnancy or calling the ER when Taylor couldn't breathe well, only to realize she had a big booger in her nose. I can admit we panicked a bit, but better safe than sorry. And that's my mantra in leading you through the steps you need to exercise while pregnant and after.

Nothing is more important than your own safety and the safety of your child. But that doesn't mean that your workout should be easy-breezy. If you work out a lot you should be able to sustain most of your workouts, but now is definitely not the time to kick it up a notch! Most doctors recommend that you work at a moderate to slightly difficult effort level. And I will introduce that level with the rate of perceived exertion (RPE) scale on page 14; it's better than target heart rates and heart rate monitors (more on that later).

I also have no doubt that you may be thinking about sagging breasts, cellulite, and stretch marks. Or even the weight gain that might have stuck around by the time your baby is a year old. Well, I am here to tell you that you can battle most of these things by simply working out during your pregnancy—and sticking with the recommended weight gain, not packing on sixty pounds.

My intention in this chapter is to not overwhelm you with information about pregnancy and fitness issues. You've got (or will soon have, in the case of those of you who are not yet expecting) enough going on in your body and your brain. But I do want to make sure that you are prepared for and have a basic understanding of some principles related to pregnancy and exercise. I also want to explain some of the myths out there about pregnancy and exercise and give you a bit of a motivational pep talk to help get you under way. Getting you motivated when all you want to do is sleep and you don't mind getting a little chubby is important. A big belly is good, but I also want you to know how much is too much. But also know you can always get that body back and that most of you will find an even better body—better than the one you had in high school!

Precautions

Please note that this book is intended for women who are experiencing normal, healthy singleton or twin pregnancies. You must consult with your doctor before you begin any portion of this program and be completely honest in discussing with him or her any possible conditions you may have or that run in your family. Because the number of twin deliveries rose by nearly 50 percent from 1980 to 2005,[5] I include some material specifically for singleton and twin pregnancies. But whether you're having or have one or two children, you must get your doctor's permission before using Part I, II, or III in this book.

> **Trying to get pregnant? Healthy nutrient storage and proper weight are just as important before pregnancy as they are during pregnancy.**

Remember when you were a kid going on a field trip and you had to have a parental permission slip signed? Consider this your *prenatal* permission slip.

I want you to sign in the blank space, indicating that you have gotten the green light from your doc to go ahead with this program:

X_____

Why You Should Exercise During Pregnancy

The fact that you have this book in your hands means that you're already interested in staying fit.

Why should you work out now? If you do, by the time your baby is a year old, your non-working-out friends will have three times more weight and two times more fat than you, and their abdominal tone won't be nearly where yours will be.[6]

Do you have the mentality of "I'll deal with it after I have the baby?" Let's talk about this. That means after three babies you could be thirty or more pounds overweight simply by having not worked out. Which brings us to:

Rule #6: Lose the Weight Between Babies! Of course, it's never too late. But I am guessing if you bought this book you are motivated to work out. And you're only going to get older and busier as your family grows, so take it in stride. Stay motivated not only for your body, but for your baby too!

Not everybody enjoys exercise like I do. So let me give it to you straight.

Rule #7: Not Exercising for Nine Months Sets You on a Long Journey to Getting Your Shape Back. You will have to start from scratch if you don't exercise for the next nine months. To push you over the edge and truly convince you that you will benefit in so many ways, I put together this list to motivate you to put my program into practice:

1. Your healthy baby starts now.
2. You can get back to your pre-pregnancy weight quicker! Working out now creates muscle memory for afterward—that's why fit people get their body back quicker.
3. You will have more energy!
4. You will experience a decrease in these pregnancy-related symptoms: back pain, constipation, fatigue, insomnia, nausea, swelling, urinary incontinence, and varicose veins.
5. Your circulation will improve, meaning you will experience less swelling—which you will be so happy with by your third trimester!

FINDING YOUR MOTIVATION

Yes, your baby is going to need food, shelter and a lil' love. But he or she is also going to need a healthy environment to grow up in. Sure, genetics plays a small role in being overweight, but your environment plays an even bigger role. When you picture your family, do you imagine them outside together at a park? Or inside playing video games, eating chips and dip?

For right now the baby's environment is your womb. So why not make it the healthiest place possible? It's the best reason to be on top of your game. And once the baby arrives you will be healthy enough to enjoy all the activities. Some moms have trouble just getting on the floor to play with the baby. Don't be ones of those.

You can't do anything about yesterday or the day before. Forget that you threw in the towel after five minutes on the treadmill or after you ate one too many Girl Scout cookies. Start now—you can do a lot about your future!

And what are the top three reasons moms work out?

1. For their kids
2. For their confidence
3. For a mood boost

6. You will deposit less fat and limit your weight gain. And like I said before, your friends who didn't exercise during pregnancy will have three times more weight retention when baby is one year old.
7. You will enjoy a quicker postpartum recovery, and usually an easier labor.
8. You will feel better in general and feel better about yourself (for which your partner will be thankful).
9. Your chances of resuming your pre-pregnancy fitness levels will be twice as good compared with those of non-exercising pregnant women.[7]
10. If you don't put this program to use, you are more likely to retain some of the baby weight. So if you keep ten pounds of baby weight after each of three children, that's an extra thirty pounds!

Step by Step

To begin enjoying these benefits, you have to take the first step. Have you ever run a marathon? Well, get ready! Being pregnant for nine months is definitely no quick sprint. I've run a marathon, and it wasn't until after I'd done one that I met another, more veteran runner who told me that it is impossible to keep an entire marathon in your head. It's just too long a race to be thinking about the whole thing. It was too overwhelming.

I have to admit that, while I was grateful for the people who lined the marathon course to cheer us on, at mile three I wanted to ask the people who were yelling, "Good job! You're almost there!" if they were serious. We still had a little more than twenty-three miles to go! I don't care how math impaired you are, three is *not* almost twenty-six.

With this lesson in mind, and knowing that most women—let alone pregnant women—can't accurately visualize what their life is going to be like in nine months, I adopt the same trio of three-month divisions (trimesters) for my program that doctors do for pregnancy and fetal development. I don't do this arbitrarily; I do it because the changes your body and your developing child are undergoing will dictate what you can and can't do, should and shouldn't do, at that particular stage in your pregnancy. And I added which weeks are within which trimester, since we are used to our doctors expressing pregnancy in weeks.

No matter which of the three phases of my program you are in, here are some guidelines that you need to follow:

1. An hour before you exercise, eat a snack of protein and carbohydrates.
2. Drink about a cup (eight ounces) of water for every fifteen minutes of exercise. This is in addition to your daily fluid intake covered in Chapter 2: Pregnancy and Nutrition 101.
3. Do not exercise for longer than fifty minutes.[8]
4. I recommend exercising three to five times a week, while doing activities such as walking, playing, housework, gardening, and the like on the other days.
5. Exhale on the effort of each exercise. You must breathe to get oxygen to that baby!
6. Your body is smart—it bears a child!—so listen to it. Do only what you are comfortable with. There is no one-size-fits-all exercise for pregnant women, and you'll be more tired on some days than on others.

7. If you are just beginning exercise, you need to refer to page 74.

8. Each trimester, the way your body, especially the circulatory and respiratory systems, reacts to exercise and other things is different, which is why each workout is broken into trimesters.

9. Try to be consistent with exercise; don't work out sporadically. Of course, it is OK to skip a day, but a haphazard approach will produce haphazard results. Consistent effort will pay consistent dividends.

10. If diastasis recti (a separation of the right- and left-side muscles of your belly) occurs, then you should stay away from twisting motions and crunches. I provide modifications to my program for those of you who have to deal with this common problem. You can also see my YouTube video to determine if you have the condition by going to youtube.com/momsintofitness.

11. If you have a moderate exercise routine, keep it up! If you have been sedentary, don't suddenly start an aggressive exercise routine, but adapt slowly. And exercise veterans should be able to sustain the same amount of working out.

12. No contact sports!

MAKING CERTAIN YOU EXERCISE SAFELY

The Big Five

1. Drink a cup (eight ounces) of water every fifteen minutes and eat an hour before starting exercise.
2. Exercise in a cool, well-ventilated area—especially important in the first trimester. Avoid hot, humid environments.
3. Listen to your body and exercise within *your* 5–8 range. (Please refer to the RPE scale on page 14.)
4. Wear good, supportive shoes to help prevent flat feet, which women tend to get during pregnancy. Wear a supportive bra and cool, dry clothing.
5. Be aware of when to stop exercising. (Refer to the list on page 14.)

Steps to Take Now for a Better Body After Baby

Believe it or not, there are moms who are more fit after having a baby than before. Your body has to work so hard during pregnancy—even without exercise—that when you add exercise to the equation, your VO_2 max, blood volume, and muscles work even harder, improving your overall fitness. Then, after the baby is born, your fitness level can remain elevated. Professional runners have demonstrated this by achieving better times after becoming mothers. So take advantage of it—pregnancy exercise is your own marathon training, without the effort.

Few women like the feeling that comes with weight gain. With pregnancy, that weight gain is inevitable, along with several other changes to our bodies. With exercise and good nutrition, you will get your body back in nine months or less, guaranteed. And most of the time it can happen in five months or less. After delivery, your uterus, which is a muscle, will return to normal size within six weeks. Without exercise, everything will slowly fall back into place and you'll be left with loose muscles—particularly around your belly. Many women want to lose their baby weight and the stomach pooch, fupa, mom apron, pudge, and every other disgusting word that goes with it. Don't worry, with my program you will. I will teach you how to use your transverse abdominis to pull your abs in tight. We will go over these transverse exercises—the only way to a flat stomach—during pregnancy and after.

Why Do Core Training?

As your belly expands, it may seem counterintuitive to work on strengthening the muscles around the area that increases in size as a natural part of pregnancy. Before I explain why this is not counterintuitive, let me tell you what the core is. As simply as possible, your core is defined as all the parts of the body except for your limbs and head. We'll get into more specifics later, but for now, think of your core as your abdomen, chest, back, and hips. Some of your abdominal muscles, in particular your pelvic floor (PF) and transverse abdominis (TA), are involved in labor. Making those muscles as strong and flexible as possible during labor greatly eases your baby's entry into the world, and you'll be grateful for that. Post-pregnancy, your healthy muscles will bounce back more quickly from labor. Your transverse acts as a sling[9] to hold that baby in! So we've got to keep it strong.

The core exercises I have you do will focus on the pelvic floor and the transverse abdominis but will also help strengthen your back—a frequent sore spot for pregnant women. Strong abs and back muscles will help ease the strain on your spine as well as on other parts of your body. Every part of you is connected, so getting those essential parts in good shape will have overall benefits as well.

The Stretch and Bubble

After pregnancy, you can be left with loose skin, stretch marks, and/or cellulite. Stretch marks are genetic in their origin, so if your mom had them, you might too. The only way you can prevent stretch marks is to watch your weight gain and make sure you gain steadily, not sporadically, during pregnancy. No creams can penetrate the skin deep enough to get rid of stretch marks or cellulite. Only exercise can reduce the amount of cellulite you have during pregnancy; strength training can even eliminate it. Remember, there is nothing you can do to improve your genetics, so it's up to you to exercise and get rid of that cellulite. Or prevent it, which is what you can do with this program.

After-baby weight loss will help you get rid of stretch marks and cellulite. As for the loose skin—your genetics, age, and skin elasticity will determine how quickly it will tighten up again. And I sound like a broken record, but if you take care of yourself during pregnancy you will more than likely eliminate any loose skin after baby. So exercise during pregnancy and you will reduce the likelihood of stretch marks, cellulite, and loose skin post-baby! Toning is especially important. More on that in Part III.

To a great degree, your genetics determines to what degree you will have stretch marks or cellulite, but that does not mean you will be overweight. You are in control of your own body.

A Brief Look at the History of Pregnancy and Exercise

Most likely, you and even your mother are too young to remember the days when pregnant women were seldom seen in public. The perception back in the day was that a woman who was pregnant was in a fragile state and needed to do everything she could to protect her health and her child's development. So she stayed home. Doesn't sound too bad—who doesn't want a reason to stay home and do nothing?

While that view of women and pregnancy has changed, there are still some remnants of that idea of pregnancy as a health condition that reflect on people's attitudes toward pregnancy and exercise. The whole "you're eating for two now" and "don't strain yourself; I'll do that for you" attitude is still quite prevalent. Pregnant women were so often viewed as helpless and needy that it took a long time for the general population to get used to the idea that women could be carrying a child and a bag of groceries at the same time.

Because America's fitness boom really didn't take off until the seventies and eighties, and the so-called women's liberation movement didn't hit its stride until about that time, women in general didn't exercise. Or at least that was the way the fitness industry and academic programs such as exercise physiology treated the subject. Sure, there were female athletes, but the general population didn't include women who worked out. It took women like Jane Fonda and Suzanne Somers to really bring exercise to the masses. As a young girl, I idolized Denise Austin and wanted to create a fitness program and empire just like she had.

Of course, things were different in my house, because my mother was a fitness instructor, but in most other households, the only kind of working out women did was for appearances. Today it might seem laughable, but in the sixties women used motorized exercise belts that vibrated and rotated the fat around their butts and hips. The thinking was that jiggling all that fat would loosen those deposits and they would somehow dissolve or burn off. (Those inventions actually made it to infomercials in 2000; FYI, they are a waste of money!)

Even once exercise among women became more popular, the accepted wisdom was that if you were a woman who worked out, you simply got sent to the sidelines for those nine months. It was as if your work was done: Congratulations! You got pregnant. Your genetic imperative has been met, so go sit over there, put your feet up, and we'll check back with you when you successfully complete the mission.

I'm exaggerating, but not a whole lot. As the women's movement proved that we are far more capable than we were once led to believe, exercise became just another of the activities a do-it-all woman was expected to be able to perform.

Still, pregnancy and exercise was a seldom talked about or examined subject in general and in college and universities as well. Studies were few and far between in the eighties; therefore, many women were told to sit and knit.

In 1985, the American Congress of Obstetricians and Gynecologists (ACOG) came out with a set of guidelines for exercise and pregnancy. And unfortunately some health-care professionals still follow them. Here are the 1985 guidelines:

- Maternal heart rate should not exceed 140 beats per minute. Note: This restriction does not appear in the 1995 guidelines.
- Strenuous activities should not exceed fifteen minutes in duration.
- No exercise should be performed in the supine position (on your back) after the fourth month of gestation is completed.
- Exercises that employ the Valsalva maneuver* should be avoided.
- Caloric intake should be adequate to meet not only the extra energy needs of pregnancy but also of the exercise performed.
- Maternal core temperature should not exceed 38 degrees C (100.4 degrees F).

Before I comment on these outdated recommendations, let me remind you of something. Trust in your doctor is essential. I am not a medical doctor and my program does adhere to the most recent guidelines established by the ACOG. I strongly believe that you should follow your doctor's advice. For those of you who are not yet pregnant and are looking for an ob-gyn, asking questions about prospective doctors' views of pregnancy and exercise, what their specific recommendations are, and which set of ACOG guidelines they follow will help you decide if that doctor is right for you.

Has someone told you that when pregnant you should keep your heart rate below 140 beats per minute? Yep, that's from the 1985 study and has since been updated. The 1985 ACOG recommendations of less than fifteen minutes of exercise and keeping your core temperature below 38 degrees Celsius were removed in 1996. Recent studies show that thirty minutes or more of exercise on most days of the week is best. And women who exercise can regulate their core temperature better than those who don't. But do not dismiss your doctor's recommendations, which may be specifically for you; you need to listen to them. Especially if you are carrying more than one baby.

---

* The Valsalva maneuver involves forcibly exhaling without allowing air to be pushed out through your mouth or nose. This is incorrect breathing for any of the exercises you will do.

Here are the most recent ACOG general guidelines:

- After the first trimester of pregnancy, avoid doing any exercises on your back.
- Avoid brisk exercise in hot, humid weather or when you have a fever.
- Wear comfortable clothing that will help you to remain cool.
- Wear a bra that fits well and gives lots of support to help protect your breasts.
- Drink plenty of water to help keep you from overheating and dehydrating.
- Make sure you consume the daily extra calories you need during pregnancy.
- Thirty minutes or more of moderate exercise on most, if not all, days of the week is acceptable for pregnant women without medical complications.
- Start exercise with a warm-up.
- Take a break when needed and never exercise to exhaustion.
- Follow exercise with a cooldown of five to ten minutes to return your body to normal state.
- Avoid motionless standing.
- Do not participate in contact sports, skiing, scuba diving, or any extreme sport.

As you can see, they removed the information about heart rate and core temperature. Here is why the 140 BPM figure is no longer used: It should not be assumed that all pregnant women working at 140 BPM are putting out the same amount of effort. **Do not use heart rate monitors, as they are inaccurate during pregnancy.**

Heart Rate and Pregnancy

Your heart rate response changes throughout gestation. It increases in early pregnancy due to underfill, then falls gradually but continually throughout the latter trimesters.[10] So, what is underfill? When you're pregnant, you're not circulating blood just through your own body, but through your baby's body. Underfill is the condition that occurs when you have a lower volume of blood pumping through your heart than you do when not pregnant. Because there is less volume going through your circulatory system with each beat of your heart, you heart rate speeds up to compensate. If you exercised at a non-pregnant woman's target heart rate, which we will use after-baby, throughout each stage of pregnancy you could easily underwork or overwork. We'll talk more about heart rate issues in later chapters.

The American College of Sports Medicine (ACSM) recommends using "rate of perceived exertion," or RPE, rather than heart rate, to measure how hard you're working. I have included my version of the scale below. The American Council on Exercise (ACE) recommends staying between 5 and 8 and ACSM recommends between 3 and 7 on a 10-point scale.[11] I have evaluated all and combined them for my scale, on which you should stay between 5 and 8.

PREGNANCY INTENSITY SCALE

0	Easy	The feeling you get when sitting
1		Activities such as getting dressed
2		The feeling you might get while doing laundry
3		Taking a casual walk
4		Walking briskly, but still maintaining conversation
5	Medium	The feeling you get when rushing out the door
6		The feeling you get when rushing up a flight of stairs
7		You are able to exercise while singing
8		Slightly tiring exercise, but you're still speaking full sentences
9		Feeling fatigue; breathing hard
10	Maximal	All-out exercise; could not maintain for more than thirty seconds

Please stay between 5 and 8.

When You Shouldn't Exercise

According to ACOG guidelines, you should stop exercising and consult with your health-care provider right away if any of the following occur:

- Vaginal bleeding
- Preterm labor
- Uneven or rapid heartbeat
- Decreased fetal movement
- Dizziness or faintness

- Headache
- Increased shortness of breath
- Chest pain
- Calf pain or swelling
- Discomfort
- Amniotic fluid leakage
- Uterine contractions that continue after rest

Always keep in mind that you know your body and your baby better than anyone, so listen to your body's cues. Here is a list of reasons why doctors may not want you to exercise while pregnant:

Incompetent cervix, multiple gestation at risk for premature labor, persistent second- or third-trimester bleeding; placenta previa after twenty-six weeks; premature labor history; ruptured membranes; pregnancy-induced hypertension (preeclampsia); significant heart or lung disease; severe anemia; unevaluated arrhythmia; chronic bronchitis; poorly controlled type 1 diabetes; extreme obesity; extreme underweight; intrauterine growth restriction; heavy smoking; poorly controlled hypertension, seizure disorder, or hyperthyroidism; orthopedic limitations.

> If you have gestational diabetes, contact your doctor about exercise and nutrition guidelines. More than likely you can follow my pregnancy workout, but your dietary habits may be different.
>
> If your doctor tells you not to exercise, then you simply have to wait until after the baby is born and follow the post-pregnancy program I've developed.

Exercise and Twins

When you are carrying twins, the demands on your body are different than when you are carrying a singleton. As a result, I have a modified program for mothers of twins. If you have a twin pregnancy you must start with the second trimester workout and move to the third trimester workout on or around thirteen weeks. Some doctors recommend that women with twin pregnancies stop working out after twenty to twenty-four weeks because they are at full gestation size around twenty-eight weeks and therefore at risk for preterm labor. And more than likely you should not do core workouts if you are pregnant with twins, especially if diastasis recti is present.

ACOG suggests that women carrying multiples should refrain from aerobic exercise. So I have adjusted the workout for you. But, again, do what your doctor says is best, which could be swimming or prenatal yoga only.

So, if you are carrying twins, get special permission from your doctor. You may or may not have permission from your doctor to exercise while pregnant with twins. And if you are pregnant with more than two babies, *do not* follow this program.

How Your Body Will Respond to Exercise

I'm still amazed every time I look at my kids and think that they lived inside me for nine months! There are times when I think it couldn't have happened, but I know it did and has been going on for thousands and thousands of years. We have evolved in such a way that every cell in our bodies adapts when we are pregnant; our bodies were made for it. Have you ever wondered why we always have a little fat below our bellies? Because we're made to bear children. While some of the changes are visible—the swelling of our bellies, enlarged breasts—many of the changes take place at a level we don't notice. We may notice the effects of those changes, but we might not understand what is going on in our bodies to produce those effects. Some are good and some are not as good, but exercise will make the good effects better offset the negative effects of the not-so-good ones.

If you're pregnant, I don't have to tell you that your hormonal balance is out of whack. That's a natural part of your body's process, as all kinds of chemical changes are taking place. The good news is that exercise is a natural stress reducer. If you exercise and benefit from the relaxation, it will also make it easier for you to sleep. If you sleep better, then the crazy hormone fluctuations are less likely to be complicated by your being cranky from lack of sleep.

Sleep is something your body will crave during pregnancy. So if you can, lie down and rest for at least twenty minutes when your body tells you it's tired. And if you battle insomnia like I did, find a bedtime ritual to help you get your z's. I found a bath, warm cocoa, reading, or the relaxation CD I got for the baby helped me drift off to sleep. And most of the time I just needed to de-stress, so I always kept a pen and paper by my bed to write down all my thoughts and to-do lists so I could unclutter my mind.

Among those changes that directly relate to exercise is the dramatic increase in the volume of work your circulatory system (heart, arteries, and veins) is doing. As a result, your body is really never at rest while you are pregnant, which is why you reach your energy/intensity level much quicker during exercise.

Your blood volume and your blood flow increase. That's why pregnant women are said to "glow." In my case, I didn't glow so much as I had a blotchy red face. Along with all those circulatory system changes, your blood pressure changes. In the early stages of pregnancy it will increase and then decrease. Obviously, a too high or too low blood pressure number needs to be addressed by your doctor, but exercise helps to even out that swing.

One of the reasons why many elite-level runners have run faster times following pregnancy is that your heart and lungs have to adapt to the increased load they are carrying. Your VO_2 max—the maximum amount of oxygen your body can process in a given time period—will increase. We most often think of this as our lung capacity. Just being pregnant (even if you don't exercise) requires you to get more oxygen (O_2) to the baby, therefore making your VO_2 max better, especially in unconditioned women and during the second trimester.[12] When you exercise during pregnancy, you boost your VO_2 even more, which increases your fitness level greatly.

One of the ways elite athletes and other very fit people keep track of whether they are working out too much, too little, or just right is by tracking their resting heart rate. The normal resting heart rate for a healthy person is around 60 BPM (you find this by averaging three mornings of counting heart rate for one minute before you get out of bed). Exercise helps lower your resting heart rate; the lower, the better. Fit pregnant women can safely work out at a higher target zone, although this zone changes as pregnancy progresses. You get to that zone a lot easier as you get bigger. Later in your pregnancy it is easier to get "winded" since your body is already working hard to support more baby. Working out will reduce stress on the heart. Remember that heart rate monitors are inaccurate during pregnancy and exercise.

A pregnant woman will experience an increase in her body's normal core temperature. Exercise also increases your core temperature, so just as you need to be careful about overheating in a sauna or whirlpool bath, you need to take precautions about not overheating while exercising. The good news is that as a result of being pregnant, your body does adapt and your ability to regulate your internal temperature improves, which is why the 1985 guideline from ACOG on exercise and core temperature was removed.

The placenta is the lifeline that exists between you and your baby. Because it is made up of blood-carrying tissues, its efficiency increases with exercise. Think of the placenta as a muscle that develops on the body—when it is in better shape, its veins grow larger and blood flows more efficiently. This is what happens to your placenta when you exercise while pregnant.

Your resting metabolic rate increases by 15 to 20 percent.[13] (Yippee! That means we can eat more!), especially as your baby gets bigger. We'll talk more about metabolic rate in Chapter 8 but for now, think of your metabolic rate like your car's engine. When your car idles, it burns less fuel. The higher the idle, the more fuel the engine burns while at rest. The same is true of your body when you are resting while pregnant. You are actually burning more calories just sitting than you did before you were pregnant.

> When you're pregnant, fat becomes a primary source of fuel for you. You convert that fat into carbohydrates for your baby. As a result, it is very important not to be on a low-carb diet while you are pregnant or trying to get pregnant, and you should eat every few hours. So if you are overweight before you get pregnant, your baby will act as a sort of "fat-burner."

Because of the extra weight you are carrying and the redistribution of that weight, some changes to your posture may occur. Lordosis (commonly referred to as "swayback") and kyphosis (hunching forward) both involve an improper alignment of the spine. My workout program targets reversing these bad postures so you benefit post-baby and don't end up with back pain. Women who work out while pregnant are about 40 percent less likely to experience back pain.

> It is important to eat every few hours while pregnant, whether you are exercising or not.

Two of the most frequent complaints that pregnant women have are varicose veins and swelling. Most of you never knew varicose veins ran in your family until you got pregnant and wondered what the heck was growing on your leg. The good news about those is that when you exercise, you increase blood flow to all the tissues in your body. That increase and stimulation of blood flow will help reduce swelling and prevent the formation of varicose veins.

The Effects of Exercise on Your Unborn Child

One of the reasons why historically women weren't encouraged to exercise was because of the possible damaging effects on the unborn child. Recent studies have shown that moderate exercise in most cases not only doesn't damage the child but actually benefits him or her. One of the major concerns had to do with the heart rate of the fetus when the mother exercised. Studies have shown that fetal heart rate does increase during the mother's period of exercise; however, that increase does not affect fetal respiration. The baby is still getting enough oxygen while you exercise. Its heart rate may increase just because of the level of activity you're engaging in. Since you are moving around, the baby is moving around as well. That disruption of normal orientation in the womb may produce a mild stress. If your baby is more active after exercise, that is normal. In fact, some researchers have discovered that babies who have been exposed to the mild stress of exercise are better able to handle the more strenuous effects of childbirth. Think of this as having your baby go through a warm-up routine before he or she actually exercises![14]

Just a reminder to all you veteran exercisers:

Oxygen is the energy for your muscles and your baby. Do not hold your breath while exercising. Try to exhale on the effort. For example, exhale as you crunch, or as you stand up out of a squat.

Are you pushing your workout? Remember, when you exercise, your muscles need blood. The uterus is a muscle and receives blood as well. Your body is amazing in adapting to keeping your baby and body supplied with blood (which carries oxygen) at all times. But if you are pushing too hard you could be sending more blood to the wrong muscles!

Studies have also shown that women who exercise while pregnant show no increase in the incidence of infertility, spontaneous abortion, ectopic pregnancy, congenital abnormalities, or late placenta complications. Also, there is no significant correlation between babies being born prematurely and the mother's level of exercise. Interestingly, one recent study showed that babies born to exercising mothers enjoyed two other benefits: They had a lower percentage of body fat and by age five they had significantly better language acquisition than those born to non-exercising mothers. Non-exercising pregnant women produced children with similar motor, integrative, and academic readiness skills, but the language acquisition skills were better for the children born to exercisers. More research needs to be done, but one theory is that exercising mothers are more relaxed and consequently more patient. Also, mothers who exercise after pregnancy frequently leave their children with others to care for them. As a result, those children are exposed to a variety of other people and stimuli, so that may help them develop their language skills. I like to think my daughter's rhythm also came from all my dancing and aerobicizing to music!

Getting Started—the Basics

Determining your body mass index (BMI) is important as you begin; it gives you some baseline information in order to figure out how much weight you should ideally gain during pregnancy. Unfortunately, just climbing on a typical scale isn't enough. Experts now rely on a different measure to determine healthy body types. The body mass index is a more accurate picture of your level of fitness and health.

So what exactly does your BMI tell you about your body and your fitness level? Along with knowing what your height and weight are, it's important to understand the correlation between the two. Simply put, your body mass index is a number that reflects the relationship between your height and weight. According to the Centers for Disease Control, if you have a body mass index of 24 or less you are at a healthy weight. If your reading is less than 18.5, you'd be considered underweight. If your BMI is between 25 and 29.9, you are considered overweight. A BMI over 30 puts you into the obese category. Individuals who fall into the BMI range of 25 to 34.9 and have a waist size of more than 40 inches for men and 35 inches for women are considered to be at especially high risk for health problems.

To determine your BMI, do the following calculations:

Multiply your weight by 703:

_____ x 703 = _____

Multiply your height in inches by your height in inches:

_____ x _____ = _____

Divide the number from step 1 by the number in step 2:

(current weight x 703) / (height in inches x height in inches) = BMI

Here's an example of a woman who weighs 150 pounds and stands five feet five inches tall:

$$150 \times 703 / 65^2 = 24.96$$
$$\text{OR}$$
$$150 \times 703 = 105,450$$
$$65 \times 65 = 4,225$$
$$105,450 / 4,225 = 24.96$$

According to the guidelines above, she is just barely over the recommended healthy weight for someone her size. Use the table below to determine your pre- and early-pregnancy BMI status:

Category	BMI Range
Underweight	18.5 or less
Healthy Weight	18.6–25
Overweight	26–29
Obese	30 and above

Appropriate Weight Gain During Pregnancy

The table shows the number of pounds a typical woman should gain during a typical pregnancy. Keep in mind that *typical* is a very slippery, very general term. Always consult with your doctor about what the optimum weight gain should be for you.

If you find that you have gained too much weight at any point, don't try to lose it or cut out significant amounts of food. Instead, slow your weight gain by focusing on cutting your consumption by only two hundred to three hundred calories per day. I'll go into much more about nutrition and calorie needs in Chapter 2: Pregnancy and Nutrition 101.

If your BMI is not in the healthy weight range, find your healthy weight range before pregnancy and try to achieve your target weight based on that healthy range number. But most of you are already pregnant if you're reading this book, so use your pre-pregnancy weight and find your BMI to estimate how much you should gain during pregnancy. Your doctor will also give you a range.

(target BMI) x (height in inches x height in inches) / 703 = target weight

**NEW GUIDELINES FOR THE APPROPRIATE WEIGHT GAIN
DURING SINGLETON AND TWIN PREGNANCY**

Category	BMI Range	Appropriate Weight Gain
Singleton		
Underweight	18.5 or less	28–40 pounds
Healthy Weight	18.6–24.9	25–35 pounds
Overweight	25–29.9	15–25 pounds
Obese	Greater than 30	11–20 pounds
Twin Pregnancy		
Underweight	18.5 or less	Insufficient data
Healthy Weight	18.6–24.9	37–54 pounds
Overweight	25–29.9	31–50 pounds
Obese	Greater than 30	25–42 pounds

Institute of Medicine, 2009.

Eating for Two Can Contribute to Obesity

You've likely heard or maybe even said one or more of the following: "I gained sixty-five pounds during my pregnancy!" "I cannot lose my baby weight!" "I've had three kids; of course I am going to be overweight!" "I didn't have this tummy before I had children." "My children only eat fast food and I'm stuck with it."

Although there is partial truth to the statements above, I am here to guide you on the right path to consecutive healthy pregnancies. Women who enter a pregnancy overweight can become even more overweight after the next pregnancy. It's not necessarily the number of children you give birth to, but how you treat your body in between pregnancies and during each pregnancy that makes the difference between getting back to healthy and fit and not.

WHAT'S SO BAD ABOUT OBESITY?

The quick answer to that question is this: Everything. According to the Stanford University Medical Center, each year obesity-related conditions cost more than one hundred billion dollars and cause an estimated three hundred thousand premature deaths in the United States. Of more personal concern, obesity can lead to:

- High blood pressure
- Diabetes
- Heart disease
- Joint problems, including osteoarthritis
- Sleep apnea and respiratory problems
- Cancer
- Metabolic syndrome: abdominal obesity, elevated blood cholesterol, elevated blood pressure, insulin resistance with or without glucose intolerance, elevation of certain blood components that indicate inflammation, and elevation of certain clotting factors in the blood. In the United States, approximately one-third of overweight or obese persons exhibit metabolic syndrome.
- Social effects: We live in a society that praises beauty and thinness and punishes overweight. Hearing and seeing those negative messages can cause devastating blows to your self-esteem.

The point here is to be proactive. If you're not obese, obviously the answer is to not get there, and don't use your pregnancy as an excuse. If you are obese, do something about it now—it is never too late to make life-saving and life-altering changes.

If you get back to your normal, healthy body between each pregnancy, you are less likely to become overweight after your second, third, and fourth child. The best way to do this is through exercise and nutrition. If you're breastfeeding, you do have an advantage, since your body is burning more calories to produce milk. And although exercise is tough to fit into your new schedule, your body and your mind will appreciate it. Start now; it's never too late! If you're guilty of eating for two, please understand this: ACOG's "Green Journal," *Obstetrics & Gynecology,* found that women who gain more weight than is recommended during pregnancy and do not lose the excess weight within six months of giving birth are at an increased risk of being obese eight to ten years down the road. The good news is that most women lose a significant portion of the weight they gained within the first month after giving birth.

Starting Your Pregnancy Overweight

Too much weight gain during pregnancy has led to America's female obesity epidemic. Think about it—if you don't lose all the weight gained during pregnancy (which is much easier to do when you gain only the recommended amount to begin with) and you start subsequent pregnancies with ten extra pounds, where will you be in the next pregnancy? The cumulative effect continues, and it doesn't take long to get into the obese category. Take care of your body now, during pregnancy, so you don't have to do all the work later!

Ongoing research suggests if a woman is obese (over 30 BMI) during pregnancy she does not need to gain more than fifteen pounds. Some doctors even say some obese women need only gain three to five pounds. A woman can actually lose weight (not according to the scale, since the baby is growing) off her own body. The baby actually uses up some of mom's fat and protein stores. That's not to say that you should count on losing weight by having a child, obviously, but with all the associated risks of being obese, it's important that you stay out of that category so you can live a healthy life and spend as many years with your child as you possibly can.

Pregorexia: Can You Ever Be Too Thin?

At the opposite end of the spectrum are women who fall into the underweight category. Unlike with obese women, the greater risk to being underweight while pregnant is that it will affect the baby's health. In 2009 the American Dietetic Association came out with an article on women who do not gain enough weight during pregnancy. An underweight woman who fails to gain adequately during pregnancy is more likely to give birth to a baby with dangerously low birth weight. Infant birth weight is a very important sign of a child's future nutrition and health. A low-birth-weight baby is defined as one who weighs less than five and a half pounds at full term; these babies are forty times more likely to die in the first year of life than a normal-weight baby.

Underweight women need to meet their nutrition needs for minerals, vitamins, and all the other necessary nutrients, and they also need to consume enough calories to safely and reasonably gain weight. Nutritional deficiency coupled with low birth weight is the underlying cause of more than half of all deaths worldwide of children under five years of age. Underweight women need to gain about forty pounds during the course of pregnancy.

Just as an overweight woman needs to determine her BMI and calculate a target weight, so does an underweight woman. Use the formula above and get started down the road to a healthy weight. By exercising sensibly, you will be able to gain weight while pregnant and maintain the level of fitness you will need to shed any extra pounds necessary post-pregnancy.

Conclusion

We all have that skinny friend who can apparently eat and drink anything she wants. It's partly due to her basal metabolic rate (BMR), but really looking into my friend's habits, I realized she does watch what she eats. Before she got pregnant she would have a big lunch, then only snack or have a small dinner. While she was pregnant she felt guilty that she was only having a snack or small dinner, so she ended up eating three big ol' meals and by twenty weeks she was up fifteen pounds. Trust me, she still looked like Olive Oyl, only now with a little softball on her stomach, but she was not excited about her weight gain. She even got a talk from her doctor about it!

The following chapter is designed to be a general overview of health, fitness, and nutrition issues related to pregnancy. I'll be spending more time on each of these topics to make certain that you have a healthy pregnancy and a healthy baby.

· 2 ·

PREGNANCY AND NUTRITION 101

I know that for active moms, squeezing in the time to work out in the middle of car pooling, meal preparation, shopping, and shepherding life is difficult. But I also know weight control during pregnancy is key (remember rule #2 on page xviii?). There is an essential difference between dieting—a word that I don't like to use because of all the images of starving yourself and denying yourself your favorite foods—and managing your weight gain during pregnancy.

The Mental Side of Nutrition

I wanted to better understand how women could gain weight, get the proper nutrients necessary to keep themselves and their unborn child healthy, and meet the goal of gaining twenty-five to thirty-five pounds during their pregnancy. When most women commit to a nutrition and exercise program when they aren't pregnant, one of the things that helps them stick with it is seeing the daily and weekly progress they are making. They are getting thinner and more toned. They feel great about being able to fit into that little skirt or that pair of jeans they thought was going to have to be relegated to the "back in the day/back of the closet" pile. That encourages them to stick with it. All the effort is worth it because as they get smaller, they can go out shopping and buy clothes that fit the new and improved, slimmer version of themselves. Everything from sexy underwear to low-rise jeans and belly-revealing tops are toted home in bags from places like Neiman Marcus, Macy's, and Saks. With the new body comes a new hairstyle, and a mani-pedi for good measure, because what's the sense of having a hot body without all the accessories and other goodies?

Well, every pregnant woman I know has experienced the opposite. They have seen a daily and weekly increase in their weight. Instead of a pair of curve-hugging jeans, it's jeans with a stretch panel. Instead of a pair of G-string panties, the only G is for granny panties. The new hairstyle? Unwashed and tucked under a baseball cap. And for real dress-up days, one of your husband's old XXL sweatshirts and a pair of Crocs that shed tears with the extra weight they're being asked to support. Yet, we're torn and we get angry with ourselves for the pity party. Weight gain is a good thing, a great thing, a wonderful, miraculous, amazing thing! It means the baby is developing and you are advancing toward the day when you will bring a new life into the world. But what the hell is up with my belly button? And did I used to have a second chin? Those negative feelings and perceptions are in competition with those feelings of being a vessel of nature's eternal mysteries and magic.

When you're pregnant your body goes through all kinds of changes, and your hormone levels are as volatile at the stock market. Staying focused on your goal of maintaining a healthy weight gain is hard. But it is also absolutely necessary and essential. One of the things I do each year is to come up with a list of goals. I suggest that if you're currently pregnant or are hoping to be, you establish a set of goals for yourself for the next year. These aren't just health goals, but ten things you want to check off your to-do list!

Here are mine:

1. Spend more time with my husband.
2. Stop working so much and start playing.
3. Finish my book so I can play more.
4. Have a larger family.
5. Be a good mom in times of stress, and play with my kids more.
6. Finish photo albums. (This seems to be on my list every year!)
7. Take more exercise classes for myself, instead of always teaching them.
8. Go to Hot Yoga more so I can get better!

9. Make others happy, so I can be happy.

10. Learn how to cook and enjoy it!

Before you get into the rest of this chapter, I want you to write down your ten goals for the year. I'm confident that I'll be able to help you achieve at least one of them: Maintain a healthy weight gain during pregnancy or reach your target weight post-pregnancy. And you know what they say about success, don't you? Success breeds success! I have a feeling that once you achieve your fitness goals, you're going to find yourself on a roll and checking all the others off your list as well!

Eating Right

We all need to eat more healthfully. One of the great things about working at becoming pregnant (besides the obvious!) and being pregnant is that your motivation to improve your eating habits is so much stronger than it would be otherwise. Knowing that eating all your fruits and veggies (two cups fruit, two and a half cups vegetables) each day is not only making you healthier but is contributing to your child's development makes it so much easier to meet that goal. If you start out with that relatively simple goal and commit to it, you will be on your way. Preparing for a pregnancy is the best time to start.

Because I am not a registered dietitian, when I began Moms Into Fitness I wanted to be sure to get the best and most scientifically verifiable information for my clients. I have all kinds of certifications and an extensive background in exercise and fitness. As a result, I also knew a lot about nutrition, but I wanted to bring on board someone who had a similar kind of background and training. Stephanie Margolis, R.D., is a registered dietitian and member of the American Dietetic Association. Much of what you are about to read on pregnancy and nutrition is based on Stephanie's work and information derived from the American Dietetic Association.

Getting Started

Preparing for a new baby is one of the most exciting and sometimes frightening things you will go through during your life. There are many questions you may be asking yourself, such as "How will I decorate the baby's room?" "What will we name our child?" "How will I handle having three children under the age of four?" "How will my life change?" However, one of the most important questions you can ask yourself is "What can I do to ensure my baby and I are healthy?" Well, just by purchasing this book you have taken the first step. By taking care of yourself with proper nutrition and exercise you are doing your best to start your baby's life off right. The quality of the first six to twelve months of your baby's life is greatly affected by your prenatal nutritional status and diet because the baby relies solely on you for all of his or her nutritional needs.

Nutrition is the foundation of life and affects all aspects of human existence. For the baby, nutrition impacts birth weight, gestational age, his or her nutritional condition, and the occurrence of birth defects. Moms may not experience nutrition-related consequences immediately; however, not practicing proper nutrition can have lasting effects on you, including conditions such as osteoporosis, obesity, and diabetes.

I'm not going to tell you not to give in to cravings, or that you shouldn't see a spike in your hunger until around thirteen weeks. Every pregnancy is different, so I am going to help you with yours. Sure, you can have your cheeseburger, milk shake, and fries, but I will teach you how to balance that out so you stay on track in your weight gain. And maybe sometimes you should eliminate the milk shake for some good old-fashioned water.

This chapter is designed to be used in addition to the workout series. You will find how to prepare yourself for a healthy baby, what your nutritional needs are for any stage of pregnancy, and how to meet them. Later on, you'll get all the information you need to rid yourself of those unwanted post-pregnancy pounds and the cottage cheese that found its way to your thighs.

Pre-Pregnancy

NUTRITION IN THREE WORDS

With all the information out there about diet and nutrition, it is easy to become confused or even frustrated by it all. But your nutrition can be boiled down to three easy words:

Balance—Variety—Moderation

If you follow these three words, I promise that your mentality of eating during pregnancy will be an "easier" change. To begin, let's look at what each of these words means:

Balance: A healthy lifestyle is much like a balancing act, in which we must match the amount of energy we put into our bodies (food) with the amount of energy we expend each day (exercise and activity). Balance also means focusing on foods from all of the food groups: grains, fruits, vegetables, meat/protein, dairy, and fats. Eating from each of these groups allows your body to receive all the nutrients it needs to function properly.

Variety: Not only is it important to eat from each of the food groups, but it is essential to eat a variety of the foods within each group. For example, eating from the meat/protein group does not mean eating only beef; it is also important to eat eggs, chicken, protein sources like peanut butter, fish, and nuts. All of these foods provide your body with protein, but each one has its own little kick of special nutrients, such as omega-3 fatty acids found in fish.

Moderation: Portion control is probably the most important thing when looking at your current eating habits. Most of you could tell me that fruits and vegetables are excellent choices, while chips are not the best snack. If you happen to be craving salt, go ahead and have a few! (We'll talk about controlling cravings a little later.) We live in a supersize economy, so it is hard to know what a serving size really is. The easiest place to start is to read the nutrition label on the side of your food packages. Another thing you can do is flip to Appendix A in this book (page 291), where you will find examples of ways to right-size your choices.

These three keywords provide a base for any healthy eating plan. For you, the expectant mother, it is important to keep these words in mind as you read the rest of this information, which will provide you with specifics about nutrition throughout your pregnancy. In each section you will find essential nutrition information for every stage based on balance, variety, and moderation.

What you are about to read will guide you in making healthy choices for you and your baby. If you are in the pre-conception stages, you should read pages 31–35 for information vital to preparing your body for a healthy pregnancy.

Being adequately prepared for your pregnancy is helping not only yourself, but your baby too. Nutritionally, there are three things you can do in the months prior to conception to ensure that you and your baby are off to a good start: Make sure you are starting at a healthy weight, build your nutrient stores, and create a new lifestyle.

HEALTHY PRE-PREGNANCY WEIGHT

Achieving a healthy pre-pregnancy weight is important for several reasons: You will be more likely to conceive easily, you'll have less chance of miscarriage, you'll encounter fewer health risks during your pregnancy, and you'll have a higher chance of giving birth to a healthy baby. The first step to identifying a healthy pre-pregnancy weight is to break out that pen and paper—or calculator—and figure out where you are and where you need to be. A good way to find out where you are is to calculate your body mass index. Follow the steps on pages 20–22 to find your BMI.

If your BMI is not in the Healthy Weight range, the next step is to find your target weight. To set your target weight, choose a BMI in the Healthy Weight category that is closest to your current BMI. Once you have determined your healthy BMI, use the formula on page 22 to find your target weight.

Keep in mind that this gives you merely a reference for a healthy weight. If you find you are extremely underweight or overweight and you want individualized attention, it is best to speak with your health-care provider or a registered dietitian in addition to using this program.

Does your weight already fall into the Healthy Weight category? If so, skip on to the next section, Building Your Nutrient Stores. If not, keep reading; the following section offers tips for weight loss before pregnancy and the section below it outlines suggestions for gaining weight before pregnancy.

TIPS FOR WEIGHT LOSS BEFORE PREGNANCY

- **Set realistic goals.** Depending on your current weight and the time at which you would like to conceive, it may not be realistic or safe for you to lose enough weight to be in a healthy weight category. Losing 10 percent of your current weight is a good goal, but make sure to talk it over with your doctor. Dr. Robert Greene, also a reproductive endocrinologist, told me losing 10 percent can also help balance your hormones, making getting pregnant easier.
- **Focus on balancing your meals with a variety of foods in appropriate portions.** It may help to keep a food journal so you can see how much you are eating and find areas that may need improvement.
- **Notice the difference between "head hunger" and real hunger.** Are you hungry because you saw a commercial for your favorite restaurant, or does your body really need energy?

TIPS FOR WEIGHT GAIN BEFORE PREGNANCY

- **Speak with your doctor about a reasonable goal.** For your body this could mean as little as a half pound each week. It depends on your body and your doctor will give you the best advice.
- **Be sure to add healthy foods that enhance the balance and variety of your diet.** Eating foods such as nuts, seeds, oils, and avocado can add calories as well as healthy fats to your daily intake.
- **End all intentional and unintentional meal skipping.** You may find that you need to plan your meals more and eat by the clock. Eating by the clock means setting specific times when you will eat and sticking to it. If you are eating five or six meals each day, you may eat at six a.m., nine a.m., noon, three p.m., six p.m., and nine p.m. (optional). If you choose to make your last

meal at six p.m., you will want to aim to eat a meal consisting of approximately 450 to 500 calories.

BUILDING YOUR NUTRIENT STORES

Focusing on balance, variety, and moderation will help you to eat healthier; however, there is more involved nutritionally when you are planning a pregnancy. There are certain nutrients that are very important in protecting the developing baby from certain birth defects as well as ensuring the baby is off to a healthy start. There are many other important nutrients needed during pregnancy, which you will find more information about on pages 60–61; however, in this section we will focus on two: folate and calcium.

PRE-PREGNANCY FOLATE

Folate is a B vitamin occurring naturally in foods such as fruits, vegetables, and fortified grains, and is used by the body to produce new and healthy hemoglobin. Hemoglobin, a component of red blood cells, carries oxygen throughout the body in the baby and in mom. The synthetic form of folate is folic acid; it is used to fortify foods such as enriched grain products, lentils, spinach, and asparagus. You can find a more complete list of folate-containing foods on page 58. In a growing baby, folate helps to properly develop the neural tube, which then becomes the baby's spine. This occurs very early in the pregnancy, often before you even know you are pregnant. Consuming adequate amounts

---

SPINA BIFIDA

A defect in which the bones of the spine do not form properly around the spinal cord, causing the spinal cord to be pushed through the incomplete closures. This leads to the formation of tumors and other devastating side effects.[15]

ANENCEPHALY

A disorder involving the incomplete development or absence of all or major parts of the brain.[16]

---

of folate one month before becoming pregnant and during the first trimester can prevent birth defects, particularly neural tube defects. Neural tube defects occur in approximately one out of every two thousand births in the United States. These defects present themselves in the form of spina bifida and anencephaly. Shoot for four hundred micrograms in the pre-pregnancy stage.[17]

Folate is the most important nutrient to get *now*, because it is estimated

ARE YOU GETTING ENOUGH CALCIUM?

Not only do your kids need calcium; women need at least one thousand milligrams of calcium a day. Women over the age of fifty need at least twelve hundred milligrams a day. Getting enough calcium can help prevent osteoporosis. There are foods besides milk, yogurt, and cheese that pack a powerful punch of calcium:

- Salmon
- Tofu
- Green leafy vegetables
- Beans
- Sesame seeds
- Bok choy
- Almonds

Calcium-Fortified Foods

- Calcium-fortified breakfast cereal
- Calcium-fortified orange juice
- Calcium-fortified soy milk
- SunnyD with Calcium
- Instant oatmeal
- Calcium-fortified bread or English muffins
- Calcium-fortified drink mixes such as Pediasure or Carnation Instant Breakfast

By learning to read food labels, you may be able to find other foods that are fortified with calcium. Most of the information provided above is from the national Dairy Council (nationaldairycouncil.org).

that up to 70 percent of neural tube defects can be prevented by getting enough folate in your diet.[18] By law all enriched grain products must include folate—and these tend to be your best sources of folic acid. Additionally, most prenatal vitamins meet your daily folate needs; however, it is still important to get folic acid from foods.

Pre-pregnancy Recommendation: 400 micrograms (or 4 milligrams) folate per day.

PRE-PREGNANCY CALCIUM

Calcium has long been known for its ability to create strong teeth and bones, but did you know that it also assists in muscle contraction (especially the heart), regulation of blood pressure, and bolstering your immunity?[19] Calcium is found in dairy products such as milk, cheese, and yogurt. It is important to build your calcium stores anytime during your childbearing years to ward off osteoporosis (thinning of the bones) and osteomalacia (softening of the bones) later in life.[20]

Meeting your calcium needs before and during pregnancy is exceptionally important so the baby can form strong bones and teeth. Getting enough calcium is important for your health too. If you do not consume enough calcium, your baby has the ability to obtain the calcium it needs from your stores, which harms your bones and teeth.

If your calcium intake is close to the recommended amount, you may not need to take a calcium supplement; however, a supplement may be helpful if you are not a big dairy person. Talk to your doctor about which supplement is right for you.

Pre-pregnancy Recommendation: 1,000–1,200 milligrams calcium per day.

Creating a Routine

Sometimes the hardest part about creating a healthier lifestyle is the initial time and effort it takes. Planning and creating a routine is a major part of making changes. This section will provide you with tips on making these lifestyle changes, along with helpful tools to get you started.

SET YOUR GOALS

Goal setting is one of the most effective ways to get you started making changes, and it helps motivate you as time goes on. The most important thing about setting goals is to think short term and small. This means that one of your goals should not be to run a marathon by the end of the month if you are barely jogging to the end of the driveway and back. If your ultimate goal is to run a race, that is fine—just be sure that it is your long-term goal and happens after you enjoy plenty of time with your new baby. Short-term goals should focus on two or three changes you can make within the next few weeks. After those two weeks are up and you have mastered your goals, build on them by adding two or three additional goals. Here are some examples of goals that have helped others:

- Do my Moms Into Fitness video three days this week.
- Add a serving of fruit at lunch three days this week.
- Add a cup of yogurt for breakfast four times this week.

RECORD YOUR PROGRESS

This can be done in a variety of ways, including keeping a food and exercise journal and using the smiley face method. A food and exercise journal helps you to track all the foods you consume and the exercise you do, to monitor your progress. This is simple to do and can be kept in a notebook or on your computer or phone app.

PLAN AHEAD

Taking time each week to outline your meals pays off nutritionally as well as for time management. Find one day that you are relatively relaxed and plan your meals for that week. Furthermore, you may find this a good time to grocery shop. Taking a list to the store will help you avoid the unhealthy foods you may normally stray toward. Take time to cut up all of your fruits and vegetables in advance, allowing you to prepare healthy meals and snacks quickly. The second part of creating a routine is to make exercise a priority! Set aside a specific time that you will exercise, and stick to it. You can even go as far as writing down your exercise time in your daily planner. You may find that when you commit to exercising with a friend you are more likely to follow through, thus meeting your activity goals.

START TODAY!

We are all familiar with the excuses made when it comes to dieting and exercise. You may find yourself saying, "I'll exercise tomorrow when I have less to do." "I already told my husband we would eat out tonight, so I'll start my lifestyle changes tomorrow." "It's not *that* big a deal for me to be at a healthier weight." While it may seem like a lot of work now, pledging to these lifestyle changes will save you a lot of worry, money, and health problems in the future. Planning for a baby is no small thing—so commit to better health today!

Nutrition and the Next Nine Months

Congratulations! Motherhood is rapidly approaching and it is more important than ever to focus on your health and nutrition. This section aims to help you do the following:

- Gain the appropriate amount of weight healthfully.
- Figure your calorie needs during each trimester.
- Identify nutrients you need in the proper amount.

WEIGHT GAIN

One of the inevitable things about pregnancy is that you will gain weight. Many women have the mentality that they are eating for two. While this is partially correct, that does not mean eating for two full-grown adults. This section will guide you to the correct amount of weight you should gain based on your body mass index, as well as offer tips to gain the appropriate amount of weight healthfully.

The health of your baby and its weight at birth are directly related to how much weight you gain during pregnancy. Gaining too much or too little weight can lead to serious problems for you and your baby. Gaining too much weight during your pregnancy—typically more than thirty-five pounds—will lead to a larger baby, meaning a more difficult delivery. Gaining too much weight also means that it will be harder to take off the weight later on. On the flip side, gaining too little weight can mean an underweight baby, who will be at a higher risk for health problems and developmental difficulties.

So, how much weight is the appropriate amount? The amount of weight you should gain is based upon your BMI, which you figured at the beginning of this book, and/or your doctor's recommendations. The table on page 248 shows you how to find your current BMI and the total pounds you should gain.

The rate at which you gain weight is just as important as the total amount of weight you gain. Here's a breakdown from the Institute of Medicine of how much you should gain and when:

First Trimester: 2–4 pounds total
Second Trimester: 3–4 pounds per month
Third Trimester: 3–4 pounds per month

As you can see, you should gain relatively little weight during your first trimester. As a result, you should not increase your food intake by very much at that point.

In general, you will be gaining a half pound to one and a half pounds per week.

You may be asking yourself where all of this weight comes from. A majority of it comes from the baby itself (seven to eight pounds) and your increasing muscle tissue and fluid (four to seven pounds). Other sources of weight gain are from the placenta and amniotic fluid that protect the baby (three to four pounds), increased size of breasts (approximately one pound), increased size of uterus (two pounds), increased blood volume (three pounds), and finally increased body fat (five or more pounds).[21]

CALORIC INTAKE

Now that you know how many pounds you should optimally gain, how can you do that steadily and in a controlled manner? The chart on pages 39–40 indicates what your daily calorie intake should be, based on your age, weight, and height pre-pregnancy. To use the chart, go down the first column to find your height. Next, find your age range in the second column and then your pre-pregnancy weight range in the third column. Once you have reached that

Age	Height	Pre-pregnancy Weight	1st Trimester Calories	2nd Trimester Calories	3rd Trimester Calories
20–25	<5'	100–140	1,800	2,200	2,200
26–30	<5'	100–140	1,800	2,200	2,200
31–35	<5'	100–140	1,800	2,000	2,200
36–40	<5'	100–140	1,600	2,000	2,200
41–45	<5'	100–140	1,600	2,000	2,200
20–25	<5'	141–180	Seek doctor's advice		
26–30	<5'	141–180	Seek doctor's advice		
31–35	<5'	141–180	Seek doctor's advice		
36–40	<5'	141–180	Seek doctor's advice		
41–45	<5'	141–180	Seek doctor's advice		
20–25	<5'	181–220	Seek doctor's advice		
26–30	<5'	181–220	Seek doctor's advice		
31–35	<5'	181–220	Seek doctor's advice		
36–40	<5'	181–220	Seek doctor's advice		
41–45	<5'	181–220	Seek doctor's advice		
20–25	5'–5'5"	100–140	1,800	2,200	2,400
26–30	5'–5'5"	100–140	1,800	2,200	2,300
31–35	5'–5'5"	100–140	1,800	2,000	2,300
36–40	5'–5'5"	100–140	1,700	2,000	2,300
41–45	5'–5'5"	100–140	1,700	2,000	2,300
20–25	5'–5'5"	141–180	2,000	2,400	2,600
26–30	5'–5'5"	141–180	2,000	2,400	2,400
31–35	5'–5'5"	141–180	2,000	2,200	2,400
36–40	5'–5'5"	141–180	2,000	2,400	2,400
41–45	5'–5'5"	141–180	2,000	2,200	2,400
20–25	5'–5'5"	181–220	Seek doctor's advice		
26–30	5'–5'5"	181–220	Seek doctor's advice		
31–35	5'–5'5"	181–220	Seek doctor's advice		
36–40	5'–5'5"	181–220	Seek doctor's advice		
41–45	5'–5'5"	181–220	Seek doctor's advice		
20–25	5'6"–6'	100–140	2,000	2,400	2,400
26–30	5'6"–6'	100–140	2,000	2,200	2,400
31–35	5'6"–6'	100–140	1,800	2,200	2,400

Age	Height	Pre-pregnancy Weight	1st Trimester Calories	2nd Trimester Calories	3rd Trimester Calories
36–40	5'6"–6'	100–140	2,000	2,200	2,400
41–45	5'6"–6'	100–140	1,800	2,200	2,200
21–25	5'6"–6'	141–180	2,200	2,600	2,600
26–30	5'6"–6'	141–180	2,000	2,400	2,600
31–35	5'6"–6'	141–180	2,000	2,400	2,600
36–40	5'6"–6'	141–180	2,000	2,400	2,600
41–45	5'6"–6'	141–180	2,000	2,400	2,600
20–25	5'6"–6'	181–220	2,400	2,800	2,800
26–30	5'6"–6'	181–220	2,300	2,700	2,900
31–35	5'6"–6'	181–220	2,200	2,600	2,600
36–40	5'6"–6'	181–220	2,200	2,600	2,600
41–45	5'6"–6'	181–220	2,200	2,600	2,600

point, move to the right across the last three columns to find how many calories you should consume each day in each of the three trimesters. For example, a thirty-three-year-old woman who stands five feet six and weighs 165 pounds should consume two thousand calories per day in the first trimester, twenty-four hundred calories in the second, and twenty-six hundred calories in the third. **This is for singleton pregnancies without exercise.**

Now, if you exercise, you get to eat more. If you exercise regularly, i.e., three to five days a week, you should follow this chart:

Please keep in mind that this chart is based on the presumption that you are beginning your pregnancy at a healthy weight.

If you are charting your weight gain progress and you notice you are not gaining weight quickly enough or are gaining too quickly, you also need to adjust. Everyone's body is different and we all have different ratios of lean to fatty tissue, different rates of metabolism, different genetic predispositions for weight gain, and so on.

Age	Height	Pre-pregnancy Weight	1st Trimester Calories	2nd Trimester Calories	3rd Trimester Calories
20–25	<5′	100–140	2,000	2,400	2,400
26–30	<5′	100–140	2,000	2,400	2,400
31–35	<5′	100–140	2,000	2,200	2,400
36–40	<5′	100–140	2,000	2,200	2,400
41–45	<5′	100–140	2,000	2,200	2,400
20–25	<5′	141–180	seek doctor's advice		
26–30	<5′	141–180	seek doctor's advice		
31–35	<5′	141–180	seek doctor's advice		
36–40	<5′	141–180	seek doctor's advice		
41–45	<5′	141–180	seek doctor's advice		
20–25	<5′	181–220	seek doctor's advice		
26–30	<5′	181–220	seek doctor's advice		
31–35	<5′	181–220	seek doctor's advice		
36–40	<5′	181–220	seek doctor's advice		
41–45	<5′	181–220	seek doctor's advice		
20–25	5′–5′5″	100–140	2,000	2,400	2,600
26–30	5′–5′5″	100–140	2,000	2,400	2,500
31–35	5′–5′5″	100–140	2,000	2,400	2,400
36–40	5′–5′5″	100–140	2,000	2,400	2,400
41–45	5′–5′5″	100–140	2,000	2,200	2,400
20–25	5′–5′5″	141–180	2,400	2,600	2,800
26–30	5′–5′5″	141–180	2,400	2,600	2,800
31–35	5′–5′5″	141–180	2,200	2,600	2,600
36–40	5′–5′5″	141–180	2,200	2,600	2,600
41–45	5′–5′5″	141–180	2,200	2,600	2,600
20–25	5′–5′5″	181–220	seek doctor's advice		
26–30	5′–5′5″	181–220	seek doctor's advice		
31–35	5′–5′5″	181–220	seek doctor's advice		
36–40	5′–5′5″	181–220	seek doctor's advice		
41–45	5′–5′5″	181–220	seek doctor's advice		
20–25	5′6″–6′	100–140	2,200	2,600	2,800
26–30	5′6″–6′	100–140	2,200	2,400	2,600
31–35	5′6″–6′	100–140	2,000	2,400	2,600

Age	Height	Pre-pregnancy Weight	1st Trimester Calories	2nd Trimester Calories	3rd Trimester Calories
36–40	5'6"–6'	100–140	2,000	2,600	2,600
41–45	5'6"–6'	100–140	2,000	2,400	2,400
20–25	5'6"–6'	141–180	2,400	2,800	2,800
26–30	5'6"–6'	141–180	2,400	2,600	2,800
31–35	5'6"–6'	141–180	2,200	2,600	2,800
36–40	5'6"–6'	141–180	2,200	2,600	2,800
41–45	5'6"–6'	141–180	2,400	2,800	2,800
20–25	5'6"–6'	181–220	2,800	3,000	3,000
26–30	5'6"–6'	181–220	2,600	3,000	3,000
31–35	5'6"–6'	181–220	2,600	2,800	3,000
36–40	5'6"–6'	181–220	2,600	2,800	3,000
41–45	5'6"–6'	181–220	2,600	2,800	3,000

Calculations provided by the author using information from mypyramid.gov.

Also, please note that this chart is for reference purposes only and is only for use by women who are having a single baby. **If you are having a twin pregnancy, do not use this chart.** Consult with your doctor regarding your nutritional needs.

To determine how many calories you are consuming, you will need to read labels. Large companies such as Pepsi have started labeling their packages "healthy."

Later in this book I will provide you with meal and snack plans and their specific caloric values so you can better reach your calorie intake targets.

COUNTING CALORIES

Due to the expanding muscle tissue, fat, and work of the heart, your needs during pregnancy increase, and therefore you burn through more calories. Recent studies suggest you don't necessarily need to increase your calories during your first trimester, but you do during the second and third trimesters.

But any way you go about it, if you are gaining too little or too much weight at any point, you need to adjust your caloric intake!

SAMPLE 300–400-CALORIE SNACK IDEAS

- 1 cup (8 ounces) frozen yogurt; 1 apple
- 2 slices bread topped with 2 tablespoons peanut butter
- 2 slices whole-grain bread topped with 2 ounces tuna fish made with 2 teaspoons mayonnaise
- 1 cup (8 ounces) skim milk, ½ whole-grain bagel topped with 1 tablespoon peanut butter and 1 tablespoon raisins (or sliced bananas)
- A homemade grilled cheese sandwich

Instead of three hundred extra calories during each trimester, shoot for four hundred during second and third trimesters.

If you find that you have gained too much weight at any point, don't try to lose it or cut out significant amounts of food. Instead slow the weight gain down. Again, there is no need to strictly count your calories; monitoring your weight gain is the best way to determine if your caloric intake is adequate. But many women need help in this category. To suggest that you simply add, say, three hundred calories to your non-pregnant diet is assuming all women know how many calories to eat to be healthy. So our chart shows you about how many calories you should consume daily with and without exercise.

All twin pregnancies must consult their health-care provider for nutritional information.

Calories come from three groups: carbohydrates, protein, and fat. Your baby is growing twenty-four hours a day and needs enough of the right nutrients to fuel its proper growth. The following will provide you with information on each nutrient and the amount your body needs.

CARBOHYDRATES

Carbohydrates are converted to glucose in the body and are quickly and efficiently used to meet your daily energy needs. However, for the expectant mother, fat is the primary source of energy, while glucose (carbohydrates) and amino acids (protein) are used by the fetus as its primary source of energy.

Forty-five to 65 of your daily total calories should come from carbohydrate-rich foods such as bread, rice, cereal, fruit, and vegetables. This is an average of 300–350 calories for a 2,200 caloric consumption. The bare minimum you should consume while pregnant is 175 grams.[22] There is no need to count carbohydrates (or fats and proteins) but it's a great idea to read labels a few times to get a general idea. It is important to focus on fiber when you think of carbohydrate-based foods. Foods that are higher in fiber include whole grain pasta, fruit with the skin on, raw vegetables, whole-grain cereals, and whole-grain breads.

The sugar you spoon into your coffee, brown sugar, white bread, candy—those are all simple sugars. They have a simpler molecular structure, which allows them to be processed quickly. You need some of these, but keep in mind their quick boost, quickly burned-out nature. They don't last. That's why you slump after ingesting them. For that reason, experts in the medical and nutritional fields have come to refer to them as "bad carbs."

Simple Carbs = Bad Carbs = Hungry in 30 minutes

Complex carbohydrates have a more complex molecular structure; it takes the body longer to metabolize them. You don't get the same nearly instantaneous rush from them as you do with the simple carbs. Because it takes longer for the body to metabolize them, you don't get the same rush-and-slump effect. And the best part is you don't get as hungry as quickly after consuming them. You can get complex carbohydrates from whole grains, vegetables, and legumes (beans). As my friend Stephanie Young, a registered dietitian says, "You need complex carbohydrates because they add fiber, vitamins, and minerals to your diet. They also keep your blood sugar from experiencing the rapid highs and lows of simple carbohydrates. Complex carbohydrates are also usually lower in calories, saturated fat, and cholesterol. Plus, they make you feel fuller longer!"

Complex Carbs = Staying Full for a Few Hours

Fiber is key for several reasons. First, it is used by the body to soften and add bulk to your stools, allowing you to pass them easier. This is important, especially if you experience the constipation or hemorrhoids that many moms-to-be experience during pregnancy. Drinking enough fluid is another important component of preventing constipation and hemorrhoids. Second, enjoying foods high in fiber will help you to feel full longer, while providing other beneficial nutrients. Complex carbohydrates, or those high in fiber, contain nutrients such as B vitamins, vitamin C, vitamin K, iron, and folate. All of these are important to the baby and will be discussed later in this section. You should aim for the recommended twenty-five to thirty-five grams of fiber each day, gradually adding it in if you are not used to eating it. Otherwise you will cause some major bloating! The easiest way to find how much fiber is in the foods you enjoy is to read the food label.

Getting More Fiber

Although you may cringe at the word *fiber*, here are some easy ways to incorporate more into your family meals (and they don't include just broccoli and beans!). Few of us eat enough fiber, so even though you are the one who's pregnant, get everyone in your family to eat better.

BREAKFAST IDEAS

Fruits are a great idea to incorporate into your and your family's meals. Family members won't even know they're eating foods with fiber!

- Make pancakes and waffles with whole-wheat mix. You can also mix in berries, apples, or raisins for extra flavor (and fiber).
- Try whole-grain or whole-wheat toast and English muffins.
- Oatmeal is yummy!
- Mix your favorite cereal with a small amount of fiber-rich cereal.

LUNCH IDEAS

- Add a baked sweet potato to your normal salad or soup.
- Make sandwiches with whole-grain bread. Make sure whole grain is listed first in the ingredients.

- Use whole-wheat tortillas to make your lunch and the kids' lunch. Roll cheese and turkey into tortillas, and cut into pieces for kids' finger foods. Wrap chicken, romaine lettuce, tomatoes, and your favorite dressing into your tortilla.
- Use the Moms Into Fitness Kids recipes.

DINNER IDEAS

- Make baked potato skins for the kids (quarter a potato lengthwise and add shredded cheese).
- Use whole-grain pasta instead of regular pasta.
- Start with a green salad, or incorporate some greens into your meals.
- Try fresh fruit for dessert.
- Check out these kids' recipes that include fiber: momsintofitness.com/recipes
Make sure you drink your water; fiber and fluid go hand in hand.

> Not eating enough carbohydrates can cause your body to go into ketosis, which can lead to brain damage and irreversible mental retardation in your baby.

PROTEIN

When you eat protein, your body converts it to amino acids, which are needed to make new cells as well as manufacture the enzymes and hormones that regulate life. As you know, your baby is growing at an incredible rate; thus, meeting your protein needs is important for the baby to grow properly. By your second trimester you need .5 grams of protein per pound of your pre-pregnancy weight per day, plus 25 grams.[23] An easier way to calculate this is by dividing your current weight in half and adding 10–15 grams.

Protein does have the ability to be stored in the maternal tissues during pregnancy, especially in the last ten weeks. This enables the body to meet your baby's growing needs. Protein also keeps the fluid balance stabilized to reduce swelling and maintain normal blood pressure.[24]

So you say you're not a big meat eater? Many foods high in protein are not beef or poultry. Nuts, legumes, dairy, eggs, and grains contain protein that helps you meet the daily recommendation. As with all other food groups, protein-rich foods provide much more than just protein to help you have a healthy pregnancy. For example, beef also contains iron and zinc. Milk is another excellent source of protein and offers a healthy dose of vitamin D, calcium, and phosphorus.

Protein is not found in prenatal supplements, so you must meet your needs with the food you eat.[25] Most Americans do not have any difficulty eating enough protein; however, focus on getting yours from the healthiest sources, such as legumes, milk, and walnuts. Protein contains iron, which is helpful in preventing anemia (more on that later).

THE VEGETARIAN MOM

Vegetarian moms-to-be often struggle to include enough protein in their diet; however, with careful planning a vegetarian diet can be healthy and safe. The first thing to do if you are a vegetarian is to inform your health-care provider of your dietary habits. You may want to visit with a registered dietitian if you would like personalized meal planning or have specific concerns. Good protein sources for vegetarians include legumes, nuts, and seeds. The most important thing is to focus on variety and adequate calories in your diet. Vegetarians may also lack iron, calcium, and vitamin B_{12}.

Do I Get Enough Protein as a Vegetarian?

All vegetarians are concerned about their protein intake. As you move through your pregnancy and into the second and third trimesters, you will need an additional twenty-five grams per day. Where is it going to come from if you are a vegetarian? Well, any good vegetarian diet includes all kinds of good sources of protein. Tofu, beans, edamame, and soy-based meat substitutes will get you the plant-based protein you need. Don't forget lentils, peas, whole grains, and nuts!

FATS

Fat can be a very scary word for most people; however, your body depends on fats to transport nutrients, cushion your organs and joints (and now baby), and provide energy. Your fat intake should be approximately 20 to 35 percent of your daily intake. Having your high-fat favorites once in a while is appropriate if you balance those choices with lower-fat foods. This is where we go back to balance, variety, and moderation, discussed earlier. Whatever you do, focus on incorporating "good" fats into your diet.

Good fats are those that help lower your cholesterol level and aid in the development of your baby's brain and central nervous system. The last trimester of your pregnancy is the most rapid period of brain development and requires a substantial amount of good fats, specifically omega-3 fatty acids. Your body is amazing in that it has the ability to store these fats to be released and delivered to the fetus when needed.

GOOD FATS

Unsaturated fats improve blood cholesterol levels, reduce inflammation, stabilize heart rhythms, and do other good things for your body. Foods from plants, such as vegetable oils, nuts, and seeds, are a good source of unsaturated fats. Unsaturated fats come in two types:

- **Monounsaturated:** Canola, peanut, and olive oils; avocados; nuts such as almonds, hazelnuts, and pecans; and seeds such as pumpkin and sesame seeds.
- **Polyunsaturated:** Sunflower, corn, soybean, and flaxseed oils; walnuts; flax seeds; and fish. (Omega-3 fats are an important type of polyunsaturated fat. The body can't make these, so they must come from food. An excellent way to get omega-3 fats is by eating fish two or three times a week.)

A lot of us stay away from things like avocado, nuts, and olive oil. We think that they are too high in fat and therefore bad for us. That's not the case. We need mono- and polyunsaturated fats. Try these to add good fats to your diet:

- Instead of cream cheese on your bagel, try almond or peanut butter.
- Try pumpkin seeds, sunflower seeds, or almonds on your salad instead of croutons. Less than your cupped hand is a good portion.
- Sauté your favorite vegetables in olive oil instead of butter to add good fats to your day.

BAD FATS

Our bodies produce all the saturated fat we need. That's why we should avoid eating foods that contain them. Our saturated fats come mainly from meat, seafood, and whole-milk dairy products (cheese, milk, and ice cream). A few plant foods are also high in saturated fats, including coconut and coconut oil, palm oil, and palm kernel oil. Look for these oils in the ingredients list and limit your intake of foods that contain them.

VERY BAD FATS

Food manufacturers want their products to stay fresh on the shelves longer. For this reason, they began using trans-fatty acids (trans fats) in their recipes. By heating vegetable oil in the presence of hydrogen gas, a process called hydrogenation, they make the oil more stable so it won't spoil as quickly. Because they are more stable, hydrogenated fats can be reused, so fast-food companies use them to fry their foods.

Anytime you see the words *hydrogenated* or *partially hydrogenated* on a food label, it means that there are trans fats in that product. The average American eats about six grams of trans fats a day. Ideally, that should be less than two grams a day, or zero if possible. A new labeling law that forces food companies to list trans fats on the label should help you keep track of and avoid the foods that have trans fats in them. Most of the trans fats we eat come from commercially prepared baked goods, margarines, snack foods, and processed foods, along with french fries and other fried foods prepared in restaurants and fast-food franchises. The quick rule of thumb is that the more processed a food is, the better off you are avoiding it. But if snack crackers are your thing, I am not going to tell you to eliminate them; just be aware of what you're taking in.

To avoid bad fats, the Harvard School of Public Health suggests that you:

1. Use liquid plant oils for cooking and baking. Olive, canola, and other plant-based oils are rich in heart-healthy, unsaturated fats. Try dressing up a salad or spring vegetables with a delicious, olive-oil-based vinaigrette.

2. Ditch the trans fat. In the supermarket, read the label to find foods that are trans-free. In restaurants, steer clear of fried foods, biscuits, and other baked goods, unless you know that the restaurant has eliminated trans fat. Read more about how to spot trans fats—and how to avoid them.

3. Switch from butter to soft tub margarine. Choose a product that has zero grams of trans fat, and scan the ingredient list to make sure it does not contain partially hydrogenated oils.

4. Eat at least one good source of omega-3 fats each day. Fatty fish such as salmon, walnuts, and canola oil all provide omega-3 fatty acids.

5. Go lean on meat and milk. Beef, pork, lamb, and dairy products are high in saturated fat. Choose low-fat milk, and savor full-fat cheeses in small amounts; also, choose lean cuts of meat.

Focusing on adding the right fats into your diet is easier than it may seem, and you can do it with the foods you already enjoy. Here are some ways that you can cut the bad fat out of your diet:

PROTEIN REVISITED

Just like with the other two main sources of calories, protein has both a good and a bad component. Protein itself is a good and necessary part of our diet. We have to take in protein every day because unlike with fat and carbs, our body doesn't store protein. And we really do need it, because it plays an important role in transporting oxygen to our cells, among other things.

The trouble with protein for most us is that, first, we eat too much of it, and second, it doesn't exist in a pure state. By that I mean that when you eat, for example, a six-ounce chunk of beef such as a porterhouse steak, you're also getting forty-four grams of fat. That's a lot of fat! So even if you manage to eat just the right amount of protein, you might be getting too much of other, bad things. So what's a pregnant girl to do? You could become a vegetarian and avoid all meat and dairy products entirely. That would be helpful, but protein consumption is tricky. There are complete proteins, which contain all of the necessary amino acids (the building blocks of protein), and incomplete proteins, which lack some of those essential building blocks. Meat and fish are complete proteins. The proteins found in things like fruits, vegetables, grains, and nuts are incomplete. There are about twenty of those amino acids that you need, so if you aren't eating complete proteins, you will have to vary your intake a lot to get all those amino acids into your system. Why do you need all of them? Because your body uses those essential building blocks to build and modify the amino acids to create the proteins you need to stay healthy. Your body can make some of the proteins you need from scratch, but it has to have all of the parts. Some parts your body can make, and some it can't.

Break Time

That's a lot of information to consume in one sitting. Let's do a quick review and then take a break and return to nutrition in Chapter 3. Keep in mind that:

- You need to set goals.
- The ABC's of good nutrition are: Balance—Variety—Moderation
- It's never too early to start a pre-pregnancy nutrition plan that includes calcium and folate.
- You need to gain weight gradually and in a controlled manner.
- You need to know how many calories you should consume during each trimester for you and your baby.
- You should gain two to four pounds during your first trimester, with the increase in pounds (as well as caloric intake) coming in trimesters two and three.
- You and your baby need to get your calories from protein, fat, and carbohydrates.
- You and your baby must consume enough carbohydrates daily to prevent ketosis.
- You need to consume complete proteins or a great variety of incomplete proteins in order to get all twenty essential amino acids.
- You need to eat fewer bad fats—saturated fats, and any foods that are hydrogenated.
- You need to eat good fats—foods such as vegetable-based oils, nuts, and seeds.

The only sense in which you should think that you are eating for two is when you are tempted to put something "bad" in your mouth. What you eat directly affects your baby's development. You don't need to be in food prison, but you should be in food school. Think carefully about what you eat, study labels, and enjoy an 80:20 ratio of classwork to recess.

· 3 ·

ADDITIONAL NUTRITION ISSUES

In Chapter 2, I talked about some of the most important issues related to eating well and controlling your weight gain during pregnancy. I joked around a bit about what it's like to be pregnant and to see yourself undergoing changes that are transforming your body from what you wanted it to be and worked hard to get to something that is useful as a tool for carrying and delivering a baby but not your ideal body image. I do think it's important to keep a sense of humor about all of this, but I also know that your health and your baby's health are important and serious issues.

In this chapter, we're going to take a look at some of the other issues related to nutrition that we didn't cover in Chapter 2. They aren't as heavy duty as the previous ones, but they're still important. I'm trying to do in this book what I'm asking you to do during your pregnancy in regard to your eating: incorporate balance, variety, and moderation. So, as I try to mix fact and fun, legitimate concerns and don't-worries, please understand that because I've been there and done that—and got the pregnancy T-shirt to boot—I'm on your side. I also understand the fun, crazy, scary, I can't wait to get this thing out of me, I'm so blessed, the world is a beautiful place, what the hell have I gotten myself into stew (that makes me want to puke!) of emotions, sensations, and thoughts that go into bringing a new life into this world. As someone who has had to undergo fertility treatments, I think I have a pretty firm grasp on just how amazing and nerve-racking the whole deal is. In fact, my grip is so firm because every time I receive another injection I'm white-knuckling something—a doctor's table or my husband's hand. Or screaming at my husband because I have yet another bruise from the few jabs it took to get the dull needle in my stomach.

Every now and then I'm reminded that we are just learning new and important information about pregnancy and weight gain. Just the other day, I came across an article in the *New York Times* about a study conducted by the University of North Carolina, Chapel Hill. The researchers there were interested in knowing what effect past dieting history had on weight gain during pregnancy. They asked twelve hundred women a series of questions, and the findings based on those interviews were interesting to me. Most women who had a history of dieting gained more than the recommended weight regardless of what they weighed at the time they got pregnant. Underweight women with a history of dieting didn't gain enough weight. Their findings were published in the *Journal of the American Dietetic Association*. (If you're pregnant and having trouble sleeping, I highly recommend reading an article from this journal just before bedtime.) What the researchers concluded was that women with a history of unhealthy eating behaviors needed extra support to get to that healthy weight gain during pregnancy. I felt a lot better about what I have been doing in working with my clients and offering them that kind of support, and I want this book to do the same thing.

I also learned that children of mothers who gain more than the recommended amount of weight are more likely to be overweight themselves by age seven. Childhood obesity is becoming a real concern in this country, and the thought that you could set your child off on that poor path while they are still in the womb is a bit frightening. I always thought that fear was a powerful motivator—the whole fight vs. flight thing. Well, in this case, I think it's important for women to fight the urges that lead to gaining excess weight during pregnancy. We all say we want a better life for our children than the one we had, and this is the first step that you can take to do that for your child.

Leah Segedie, creator of Fitness Hangout for Moms (bookieboo.com), lost one hundred pounds in between her two pregnancies. Here's her story, in her own words:

After losing more than one hundred pounds it's been psychologically very hard to gain weight with this pregnancy. My first trimester had me very upset and restricting calories like crazy. I was just doing things normally, like I was when losing, but then realized I was going to have problems, so I added three hundred calories so that I would stop losing weight. Then the nausea started and I was dying. Not eating made the nausea worse, and eating French bread, sugary cereals, and pizza made me feel so much better. I couldn't stand to look at a lot of the healthy foods I used to eat. Things like soybeans, chicken, whole-wheat bread, and vegetables made me so queasy that I was running to the bathroom to hurl. Disgusting. After a bunch of soul searching, I decided to eat what I crave and continue to exercise hard. After speaking with some nutritionists, I learned that your body will tell you what you lack and need for the baby. (I had plenty of iron, but needed the extra glucose—i.e., sugar and refined wheat—for a while, and now my body needs more protein and lots of calcium, so I've been eating more dairy products, chicken, and hummus.)

So that is what I've been doing. I'll be at seven months next week and have gained more weight than I wanted, but less than the first time. I've been doing a lot of exercising, which has probably saved me from gaining an extra twenty pounds. And yes, I have to fight that voice in the back of my head that says, "Hey, you're pregnant now; eat whatever you want." Some days I gave in and it was ridiculous, and other days I didn't. I've been fortunate enough to crave lots of fruit and things that are good for me, but the portion control just hasn't been there.

I'm sure things were a lot simpler the first time I did it, but I had *a lot* of weight to lose, so it all balances out in the end. This time I don't have as much, but I will have more challenges. I'm looking into getting a really nice jogging stroller for two, and of course I'll have support with child care from my mom and cousin while I go to the gym or boot camp.

Only eighty-nine days to go!

Fluids

Food isn't the only thing we consume while pregnant. You need to drink at least sixty-four ounces of water a day during your pregnancy, mostly to keep up with your expanding blood supply.[26]

> A good rule of thumb for water is to drink eight 8-ounce cups a day, and if you're exercising you should add about a cup for every fifteen minutes.

Fluids such as milk and juice count toward this total; however, caffeinated beverages actually count against your total because they are diuretics—they make you pee and lose fluids. And remember that drinking water helps reduce swelling!

I know that during pregnancy you already feel a bit like a pee-processing plant, and drinking all those liquids will only add to the production levels. However, not drinking enough water contributes to fatigue, headaches, dry skin, and a whole host of other not-feel-goods. I also look at it this way: As much of a pain in the bladder it is to have to pee all the time, getting up and moving is a good thing. Of course, being in the car and having to find a public bathroom is no fun, but if you shout, "Pregnant woman coming through!" you seldom have to wait in line when you do find one.

A word about alcohol: Any type of alcohol is strictly prohibited for those who are already pregnant or who are trying to conceive. Alcohol affects the growing baby by depriving it of the oxygen it needs to correctly develop all of its organs.

SOME THINGS TO AVOID WHILE PREGNANT

- Processed and junk food
- Smoking and alcohol
- Hot tubs, saunas, and X-rays
- Raw or undercooked meats
- Processed meats such as hot dogs (or in moderation)
- Swordfish
- Shark
- King mackerel
- Tilefish
- Soft cheeses not made with pasteurized milk
- Herbal tea (still being researched)
- Caffeine in amounts over two hundred milligrams
- Recreational drugs
- Certain medications (consult your doctor about any you're considering taking)
- Changing the litter box

CAFFEINE COUNTS (MG)

Brewed tea, 8 oz	20–110
Iced tea, 8 oz	10–50
Mountain Dew, 1 can	55
Pepsi, Diet Pepsi, 1 can	37
Coke, Diet Coke, 1 can	31
Chocolate milk, 8 oz	2–8
Chocolate chips, ¼ cup	26
Chocolate ice cream, ½ cup	4–5

Vitamins and Minerals

Throughout your pregnancy, your body is going through major changes. During the first trimester, the baby is undergoing rapid cell division and growing at an incredible rate as it develops each organ. This process continues through the second and third trimesters. Your body relies on many nutrients to provide for proper development of each organ. Specific nutrients include folate; calcium; iron; sodium; vitamins C, A, and D; and a bunch of the B vitamins.

FOLATE DURING PREGNANCY

As mentioned previously, folate helps to properly develop the baby's neural tube, which later becomes the spinal cord. This happens very early in your pregnancy, often before you even know you are pregnant. Folate is also called folic acid, which is the form of folate found in your everyday foods as well as any dietary supplements.

Folate is so important for all women of childbearing age that the government requires that all enriched grain products—including most breads, flours, pasta, rice, and cereals—be fortified with folic acid. Any pregnant woman needs six hundred micrograms of folate per day—but do not exceed one thousand micrograms.[27] If you are taking a multivitamin, drinking a cup of orange juice, and eating two pieces of bread you should be meeting your folate needs.

HERE'S A LIST OF GOOD SOURCES OF FOLATE THAT YOU CAN CONSUME TO INCREASE YOUR INTAKE:

Food Source	Micrograms of Folate
1 cup fortified breakfast cereal, such as Total	800
1 cup spinach	130
1 cup orange juice	110
1 avocado	55
1 cup fortified pasta	50
2 slices fortified bread	40
1 cup shredded romaine lettuce	40
1 ounce peanuts	40[28]

Folate may not sound like something tasty, but as you can see, the foods that contain a healthy amount of it are.

It is best to try to eat your high-folate fruits and vegetables either raw or lightly steamed, because this nutrient can be destroyed by cooking.

CALCIUM DURING PREGNANCY

If you have inadequate amounts of calcium in your diet, the baby is forced to pull calcium from your bones to fuel its own development. Calcium is exceptionally important in the last three months of pregnancy, when the baby's bones and teeth are developing. You should aim to get at least one thousand milligrams of calcium each day—but not more than twenty-five hundred milligrams. This amount is equal to approximately three or four servings of dairy or other calcium-fortified foods. Since most prenatal vitamins do not provide all of the calcium you need daily, you must find calcium in foods. During pregnancy, your body has the ability to absorb more calcium than when you're not pregnant.[29] All the hormones help you absorb more calcium, but vitamin D is essential for absorption, which is why milk, which contains vitamin D, is a great way to get your calcium. You can also get vitamin D by spending a few minutes in the sunlight. Below you will find common dairy foods and the average amount of calcium in each.

Food Source	Milligrams of Calcium
1 cup skim milk	300
1 cup plain yogurt	415
½ cup 2 percent cottage cheese	77
1 ounce American cheese	174
1 ounce Swiss cheese	272
1 cup soy milk	300

National Dairy Council, 2010

Talk to your health-care provider if you don't think you are meeting your needs for calcium or folate. He or she may recommend eating Tums for calcium and/or provide a supplement for you. As mentioned earlier, a prenatal vitamin will help you get a lot of nutrients. There is not enough research on herbal supplements for Moms Into Fitness to recommend them. Most important, you should speak to your doctor about any supplement or vitamin.

There is no need to worry if you do not eat the perfect pregnancy diet every day, as long as your nutrient needs are met over the course of a few days and your weight stays in check.

IRON

Iron helps deliver oxygen to your developing baby. You need twice as much iron while supporting a growing baby—27 milligrams, to be exact.[30] You will usually be tested for anemia (a lack of iron) between twenty-four and twenty-six weeks. An iron supplement will be prescribed if you are even slightly anemic. These supplements may cause constipation or nausea. For constipation, increase your fiber intake, as mentioned previously. You should take the iron supplement at a different time than your prenatal vitamin for the most benefit.

Iron is found in vitamin C–rich foods such as tomatoes, kiwi, oranges, and strawberries. You can also find iron in fortified cereals and breads. Legumes, shrimp, and red meats have about the same amount of iron as these fortified breads and cereals. A sandwich made with whole-grain bread can have up to five milligrams of iron.

MORE NEEDED NUTRIENTS

This list covers vitamins and minerals the American Dietetic Association identifies as additional needs during pregnancy, along with the foods you can find them in.

Vitamin A: sweet potatoes, carrots, spinach, milk, liver
Thiamin (B_1): pork, whole grains, enriched grain products, lentils
Riboflavin (B_2): dairy products, enriched grains such as cereal
Pantothenic acid (B_5): yogurt, sweet potatoes, eggs
Niacin (B_3): meat, poultry, seafood, fortified grains
Vitamin B_6: poultry, fish, pork, bananas
Vitamin B_{12}: salmon, tuna, Wheat Chex cereal
(Vitamins B_6 and B_{12} have been found to be helpful in battling morning sickness.)

Vitamin C: red bell pepper, orange juice, strawberries

Zinc: oysters, Total cereal, turkey

Choline: eggs, broccoli, shrimp

Magnesium: spinach, brown rice, halibut, whole-wheat bread

Sodium: cottage cheese, soup, corn

Potassium: sweet potato, banana, halibut, white beans

Iodine: dairy products and table salt

LOW-CALORIE COMFORT FOODS FOR THOSE CRAVINGS!

- Homemade mashed potatoes made with chicken broth instead of butter or cream
- Angel food cake
- Homemade hot chocolate
- Chicken noodle soup
- Grilled cheese made with 1 tsp olive oil and low-fat cheese, served with tomato soup
- 1 cup soup from your favorite restaurant
- Sliced apples drizzled with cinnamon and 2 tsp butter, zapped in microwave for 60 seconds
- Oatmeal
- Slow-Cooker Beef Stew (see page 295 for recipe)

No matter what you're craving, you need to remember Balance, Variety, and Moderation. And don't forget everything you just read about all the nutrients and vitamins you need to pack into your day. I get full thinking of that alone!

• **Balance:** If you find that you are craving certain foods, try to incorporate another food group to balance your meal or snack. For example, if you crave ice cream, add a fruit serving with sliced strawberries or bananas.

• **Variety:** Sometimes you may find yourself craving something sweet or salty. This is when you should focus on variety in your cravings. If you crave something sweet, don't always reach for candy—try fresh fruit to satisfy your cravings. If you crave foods that are salty, avoid the chips and reach for a handful of nuts or pretzels. Another example would be if you crave chocolate, reach for a refreshing glass of chocolate milk.

• **Moderation:** Think small with your higher-calorie cravings. It is OK to have a piece of chocolate, but you do not need the whole candy bar or the entire bag of sweets.

Do We Really Know How Much Sugar We Consume?

The government requires that sugar be printed on labels in grams. We shrug our shoulders at forty grams of sugar on a can of soda. But would you think twice if you read ten teaspoons?

That all sounds great, but let's get real—you're going to have food aversions! Most aversions, or "Get that away from me before I throw up!" responses, will hopefully be gone by your second trimester. I couldn't stand the taste of chicken my entire pregnancy. But only eating beef would not do my baby or my body much good. So I added a variety of proteins by adding sunflower seeds to salads, and string cheese and shrimp cocktails for snacks. And because of its high calorie count, I limited the beef intake to three or four times a week. While I love shrimp, I ate less than twelve ounces of it per week. Grilled cheese and tomato soup was a great meal until I couldn't stand the heartburn the tomato soup gave me. But the grilled cheese had iron and protein (make sure to get iron-fortified, increased-fiber bread).

Why You Should Eat Fish During Pregnancy

With the constant media attention on not eating fish during pregnancy due to high mercury content, there is not enough emphasis on why you should eat it! Fish contains omega-3 fatty acids that are extremely beneficial to you and your baby. Fish is also rich in nutrients and high in protein while low in calories.

You will want to limit yourself to about twelve ounces per week of fish. And stay away from swordfish, king mackerel, tilefish, shark, and wild salmon. I remember this by remembering to stay away from the big fish, and only eating other fish two, maybe three times a week.

There's no doubt you're going to have cravings as well. They key is to watch it. For me it was Mexican food and licorice. So I limited myself to two drive-throughs a week. As for the candy, well, I tried (emphasis on "tried") to eat it only a few nights a week. I had to throw away supersized boxes my husband brought home (out of sight, out of mind). But then there were the Girl Scout cookies. After polishing off one sleeve of mint cookies in three days I had to get them out of the house. Sure, my family was mad, but they didn't need the pure sugar either! But a good way to detour cravings is by eating a well-balanced snack every few hours, such as an apple and string cheese, a grilled cheese sandwich, a baked potato with light sour cream, yogurt bars, or a whole-wheat English muffin with peanut butter. I know it sounds like a lot of calories, but those snacks are less calorie rich than cookies and candy. You will have to find something that works for you by trial and error. And if you want a milk shake, make sure to go to the Golden Arches—they use ice milk in their shakes, which makes them the better option when it comes to fast food.

FAST FOOD

So, am I advocating fast food while I'm also saying eat right? Well, my rule of thumb is this: Try to eat well 80 percent of the time and let yourself indulge a little the other 20 percent while pregnant. (This changes to 90/10 after pregnancy!) Most of us are not going to eat only whole-grain products or only organic products. Just be cautious in eating high-fat foods and the stuff you know you shouldn't be eating. Be conscious of what you're eating; this is true all the time, not just during pregnancy. Do not grab a snack as you pass the candy bowl and do not eat leftovers off your other children's plates.

And as for those drive-through feedings—be cautious! You can consume too many calories and not enough nutrients. Try to limit yourself to two to three times a week or less. And you don't need to supersize because you are pregnant! Your fats need to come from good sources like green beans in olive oil, not french fries!

Yes, we should skip the drive-throughs and feed ourselves and our families only the most natural, healthy foods. But is that a reality for every mom? Probably not, so here are some better options for you. This is according to calories only.

If you are not in the car, or if you live in a city where you walk everywhere, go for soup or salad (no fried toppings or full-fat dressings), Asian vegetables, or a small piece of pizza.

A DIFFERENT KIND OF "FAST FOOD"

We all know we should stay away from fast food. Not only is it high in cholesterol and fat, but it can drain your energy and add pounds to your figure.

So here's some at-home fast food:

- Light or low-fat TV dinner served with a side of vegetables
- Homemade grilled cheese and a cup of soup
- Bagged salad with light dressing and shredded cheese
- Crackers, turkey, and cheese
- Fresh soup from the grocery store
- replacement meal bar with at least 3 grams of fiber and less than 250 calories
- Drinkable soup and crackers (not the whole sleeve of crackers!)
- Next time you're at the store, stock up in the meal section. They can prepare anything from steamed shrimp to baked salmon.
- Prepare breakfast foods ahead of time.

If you can, take a salad to go. Once again, no fried toppings or full-fat dressings. That'll be my number one recommendation unless you are really, really craving a cheeseburger (get a small one).

And I am going to go ahead and tell you: no double burgers and no Whopper-sizing anything. And if you're at a burger joint, no shakes or sodas—only water, unless you plan on a small shake being your meal.

My advice on breakfast? Never, ever start your day driving through a fast-food restaurant. Pack a piece of fruit or a granola bar in your purse.

I chose these options based solely on caloric content, and found the content on each of their Web sites.

Calorie-Conscious Fast-Food Options:

Taco Bell: Two tacos (not Supreme) or a burrito, fresco-style. Getting a taco salad? Skip eating the shell and use salsa as your dressing.

Arby's: Roast beef sandwich or Arby's melt with applesauce

Blimpie: Six-inch regular turkey and provolone with mustard and veggies, or six-inch regular roast beef and provolone with veggies

Hardee's/Carl's Jr.: Charbroiled BBQ chicken sandwich or four-piece chicken stars and kids' fries

Chick-fil-A: Char-grilled chicken sandwich and small waffle fries, or chicken sandwich and fruit cup

Qdoba: Tortilla soup and soft taco, or two chicken soft tacos with light sour cream

Pizza Hut: Two slices Thin'N Crispy pizza

Wendy's: Junior hamburger with kids' fries, ultimate chicken grill sandwich and side salad, sour cream and chive potato and side salad, or large chili and a few crackers

Del Taco: Bean and cheese green burrito and side of rice, or chicken soft taco and regular taco

McDonald's: Hamburger kids' meal, small shake as a meal, or six-piece chicken nuggets

Jack in the Box: Chicken fajita pita made with whole-grain, two egg rolls and a fruit cup, or small curly fries and small hamburger

Starbucks: Café Americano, tea, Vivanno Nourishing Blends, or plain coffee with skim milk, no whip

Panera: Plain bagel with reduced-fat cream cheese, pumpkin muffin, any soup, half chicken Caesar on focaccia, or half chicken salad on whole grain

Chinese: If you are getting a Chinese chicken salad, skip the crispy strips or get steamed vegetable rolls

Your local deli: Shy away from croissants and chicken salad

Pizzeria: Stick to thin crusts and veggie toppings

Eating Organic

Eating organic simply means eating foods that were grown without pesticides. They are not nutritionally better for you or lower in calories. But if you choose to eat organic, do so with fruits, vegetables, and dairy. Eating organic is environmentally wise. By not using pesticides and genetically engineered seeds, organic farmers produce crops more naturally and with renewable resources. If you don't consume foods treated with chemicals, your baby won't ingest those chemicals, and American farmers use *a lot* of chemicals. It is always wise to rinse your fruits and vegetables before eating them, but it is even more important when you are pregnant and later when you breast-feed. Look for Certified Organic on the label—that means the products were grown and processed according to standards set by either a state or private organization. Get to know your local store's produce manager, or better yet, go to a local farmers market and get to know the men and women who produced the crop of organic produce you buy!

Other Food Facts

SOFT CHEESE

Brie and feta should not be consumed during pregnancy, unless they're made with pasteurized milk. Most cheeses in the U.S. are made with pasteurized milk and are therefore considered safe. Make sure to check the label on any dairy product to ensure that it is pasteurized. If going organic on the dairy stuff, check the label as well. You don't want to take any chances on ingesting bacteria that your immune system won't be able to fight off.

DELI MEATS

The verdict is still out on whether pregnant women can eat a turkey sandwich. Deli meats sometimes contain listeria, a rare but potentially deadly bacteria. To get rid of listeria you must cook or steam the meat. It is also best to avoid hot dogs, all undercooked meats, and raw-fish sushi.

DHA

Otherwise known as omega-3 fatty acids, DHA is found in cold-water fish such as salmon and tuna and is beneficial for baby's brain development in the third trimester. If you are not getting enough (250 milligrams daily), ask your doctor for a supplement. DHA is also found naturally in breast milk.

Is it beneficial to eat fish while pregnant? Yes, the omega-3 fatty acids found in salmon, flounder, cod, shrimp, halibut, and so on are unique "good" fats. These good fats can help prevent preeclampsia as well as enhance the baby's brain development, especially after the twenty-fourth week.[31] Fish is also low in calories and is a great source of protein.

As with anything else during pregnancy, you should not go overboard. Limit consumption to two to three times a week and completely avoid high-mercury fish such as fresh tuna (not canned tuna), swordfish, shark, and king mackerel. And never eat raw fish or raw shellfish.

FLAXSEED

You don't like fish? Flaxseed is the best plant source of omega-3 fatty acids and is packed with fiber and other nutrients.

One tablespoon of flaxseed contains:

- 40 calories
- 1.6 grams protein
- 2.8 grams carbohydrate
- 2.8 grams fat (including 0.3 grams saturated, 0.6 grams monounsaturated, and 1.8 grams polyunsaturated fat)
- 2.5–8 grams fiber
- 3 milligrams sodium

Studies have shown that flaxseed reduces the risk of cancer and tumors in the breast, prostate, and colon as well as having many other health benefits, including lowering total cholesterol and blood pressure. It is also known to help your baby's brain and eye development while you are pregnant. Either brown or golden flaxseed is good for you; they have the same benefits, but the lighter (and more expensive) golden type is easier to disguise in food. Ground is a common way to consume flaxseed; you can also make crackers using whole flaxseed. Most doctors recommend that you can safely take in one tablespoon of ground flaxseed per day as a supplement. It's best to speak with your physician before adding flaxseed to your diet.

> Instead of going into a recipe for morning sickness, fatigue, swelling, constipation, IBS, and all the other fun things that come with pregnancy, I am going to tell you this: Exercise will help minimize most of them! There is no other one-size-fits-all solution to all the common complaints!

Keeping a Food Journal

One of the ways people successfully diet or maintain healthy eating habits is by keeping track of everything they eat and drink in a given day. I recommend that all my clients do this. I know that as a mother-to-be, you are going to have quite a hectic life, and tracking all you eat all the time is not possible. So, I'm going to give you a break and ask that you keep this journal for only three days per trimester.

Why do it at all? Well, a food journal is kind of a diagnostic tool that you can use in case you develop any problems along the way. If you are suffering from constipation, fatigue, or whatever, we can't just chalk that up entirely to hormones or just a "natural" part of pregnancy. There is a cause and effect. By keeping a food journal you may be able to figure out what is causing you to have heartburn. If one of your cravings is a Taco Bell Burrito Supreme and you notice the next day that you have heartburn, then you may need to reconsider the burrito being a part of the 10 percent of your "recess" eating. Or if you note that you eat it at two in the afternoon and you're fine and you eat it at ten p.m. and suffer, then maybe you need to modify *when* you eat rather than *what* you eat.

The other main function of the food journal is to track how many calories you are consuming. I ask you to track only three days per trimester (that works out to one day per month of gestation), but ideally, you will keep the journal with greater frequency. The people who most successfully manage their weight are the ones who track their intake regularly and honestly. Knowing what you ate, when, and how much is invaluable. If you are planning on having additional children, that food journal will serve as a valuable resource. You can consult it ahead of time to see what worked for you and what didn't, whether you managed to eat from each of the three food groups in proper proportion, whether you consumed enough water, and so on. Having a baby is a little like taking a test: It would be good to have your notes from the last one to use as a cheat sheet. And if you choose to breast-feed later on, it will be very important to keep a food journal and track your intake. (More on that in the pregnancy section to come!)

The Food Groups Revisited

I just said it's important to know how you did in eating the right proportion from each of the food groups. You might be wondering what those proportions are.

1. Grains: 6–9 ounces, including at least 3 ounces whole grains. An ingredient list starts with the word *whole*, not *9-grain* or *wheat*.
2. Vegetables: 2–3 cups
3. Fruits: 2 cups; try to avoid too much fruit juice
4. Milk: 3 cups, preferably low fat
5. Meat/beans: 5–7 ounces, preferably low fat
6. Fats/oils: 4–6 teaspoons

HOW TO GET MORE FRUITS AND VEGETABLES IN YOUR DIET

- Add fruit to your cereal, oatmeal, or waffles at breakfast.
- Go to the grocery salad bar. Use lots of dark greens and other vegetables instead of piling on all of the extras like eggs, bacon, and croutons.
- Add frozen veggies to any pasta dish.
- Keep fruits and vegetables in line of sight. Grapes, oranges, bananas, and apples make a colorful bowl arrangement on the table. If you see them, you will eat them. On that note, out of sight, out of mind on the sugary snacks.
- When cooking vegetables, make two to three times more than you need and immediately store the extra for tomorrow. It will save you time later on when you might not feel up to the task of cooking.
- If you must have pizza, load on extra veggies.
- Frozen fruit and veggies are nearly as healthy as the fresh stuff. They are packaged at their ripest point.
- Bring a frozen meal to work for lunch, and add a side of veggies from last night's dinner.

WHEN SALADS ARE *NOT* BETTER FOR YOU

Salads are good for you, right? If you are pregnant, salads are a great choice for filling up on your nutrients and fiber. And for all women, salads provide lots of antioxidants, fiber, vitamins, water, and a sense of fullness. But you need to watch what you put on your salad or you may end up eating as many calories as there are in a double cheeseburger.

Keep your salad colorful. Cover your salad with red peppers, broccoli, bean sprouts, carrots, cauliflower, cucumber, spinach, and tomatoes. All of these ingredients provide water, fiber, and a sense of fullness without too **many calories.**

Get your cheese on the side. Most premade salads contain six to twelve tablespoons of cheese. Just four tablespoons of cheddar cheese puts you over one hundred calories (or half of a kids' fries).

Use your palm to measure protein. For poultry, meat, eggs, and fish, use your palm to measure one serving. This adds up to 150 to 300 calories.

Measure your beans, nuts, and seeds. One tablespoon of sunflower seeds has about eighty calories, while a quarter cup of beans has about fifty calories.

Use the best dressings with the least calories. Try anything low calorie, Italian, or oil and vinegar for about twenty calories per tablespoon. Blue cheese, ranch, French, and the like contain about 150 calories per two tablespoons.

As you can see, it's easy for the calories to pile up to eight hundred or more for something so "healthy." Try a broth-based soup alongside a small salad for a filling meal.

Conclusion

Eating in preparation for your baby's arrival is a crucial component of overall good health for you and your baby. In addition to what we discussed in Chapter 2, here are the things to keep in mind:

Fluids: Yes. At least sixty-four ounces a day.
Alcohol: No. Not in moderation and not at all.

Folate, calcium, and iron: Don't rely solely on your prenatal vitamin. Eat foods rich in these minerals.

Food cravings: Give in moderately and count them as your 20 percent recess foods.

Food aversions: You're going to have them. Don't worry; they will usually go away, and no one is going to force-feed you any of your "pukers."

DHA omega-3s: Avoid foods that could be bacteria rich (raw eggs and fish, some deli meats).

If you eat the right amount of fiber, drink enough water, and eat sensibly and regularly, you can reduce the risk of fatigue, swelling, heartburn, hemorrhoids, and constipation. You may not be able to eliminate those problems, but in the end you can reduce their effects.

Keep a food journal to track your calorie consumption and your eating habits. Learn from your own experiences!

· 4 ·

PREGNANCY AND EXERCISE 101

Now that you're on the road toward your goal of achieving a gradual, healthy, and controllable weight gain during pregnancy, it's time to turn to the second phase of Operation Healthy Weight Gain. Speaking as General Lindsay, let me tell you that you've joined a kinder, gentler army of pregnant sisters. The idea that exercise can be helpful only if it hurts went out the door with headbands, leg warmers, leotards, and Marge Simpson–like big hair (thank God perms were only temporary). The exercises that I ask you to do in this fitness program (See how kind that is? I'm not ordering you to do anything!) were designed with two primary goals in mind: to keep you and your baby safe, and to honor the reality that you only have so much time in your busy schedule for exercise. No long-term deployments, no boot camp mentality to break you down so I can build you back up in the image that I have in mind. Now that you're pregnant, you need to treat yourself well, and that's what I intend to do.

Note this, however: There is a big difference between treating yourself well and spoiling yourself. I'm entirely sympathetic, but I'm also not a sucker. I want exercises and not excuses. Working out is exactly that—it's work. I have tried to make this program as enjoyable as can be, considering that physical exertion for some people is not at the top of their list of fun things to do.

I also understand that, just as it is true of nutrition and eating right, you won't see the same kinds of results Exercising While Pregnant (EWP) that you would if you were Exercising Not Pregnant (ENP). Toning and sculpting exercises, while important, just aren't going to produce the same noticeable effects on your body when EWP. Some of you may notice differences in, for example, some of the slack being taken out of the hammocks that swing under your arms, but that won't be true for all of you. Again, attitude is so important here, and you have to think ahead. Now that I think of it more, what you need to do is to think "a-body." Envision for yourself the shape you want to be in nine months after you deliver. All of the work that you do EWP will show up eventually. The program that I've devised for you post-pregnancy will be so much more effective if you are able to do the work while pregnant. You'll see quicker results post-pregnancy, and that will certainly make it easier for you to keep up with the program.

A More Tangible Goal

Though they weren't the first to come up with this idea, many women have commented to me on something they've seen on television's *The Biggest Loser*. The contestants on that program who get chosen to attend the actual camp are asked to bring with them an item of clothing or an outfit that they want to be able to fit into someday. I'm going to ask you to do the same thing. I know that for me, the fun of going out and buying maternity clothing wore off after a while. So you get to do some shopping for the future you. Some women I've worked with who've done this have purchased a bathing suit they want to fit into, and while that's probably the most visible (or invisible, as the case may be) choice to reveal the success of your nutrition and exercise efforts, it's certainly not the only one. The old standby of skinny jeans—and I don't mean the style but the jeans you can't wait to squeeze back into—will do as well. Whatever you choose to buy, don't stuff it into the back of your closet or armoire. Keep it someplace visible as a daily reminder of where you want to be.

Some women have kept "before" and "after" photos of themselves in a prominent place—tucked into the edge of their makeup mirror, on the dashboard of the car (a particularly effective means of curbing your drive-through habit), or on their nightstand next to the alarm clock as a twice-daily reminder of the goal they hope to achieve. Whatever you choose and however you choose to do it, be certain that you have a specific goal in mind. When you turn the pages to the exercise descriptions, you will see that every one of them has a specific set of target muscles or general fitness goals listed along with it. The more precise you make your goals, the easier it is to monitor whether or not you've achieved them.

As a quick reminder, here are the basic guidelines you should follow before you start your exercise program:

THE BIG FIVE

1. Drink a cup (eight ounces) of water every fifteen minutes and eat at least an hour before starting exercise.
2. Exercise in a cool, well-ventilated area—especially important in the first trimester. Avoid hot, humid environments.
3. Listen to your body and exercise within *your* 5–8 range. (Please refer to the RPE scale on page 14.)
4. Wear good, supportive shoes to help prevent flat feet, which women tend to get during pregnancy. Wear a supportive bra and cool, dry clothing.
5. Be aware of when to stop exercising. (Refer to the list on page 14.)

Exercise Essentials

Before we get into the specifics of the exercises and the daily routines, I want to be certain that we are all on the same page with your baseline of knowledge of exercise during pregnancy. If you are new to working out, don't worry. Nothing in here will be so technical that you'll feel like you're studying for an exam.

BREATHING 101

OK, take a deep breath. No, seriously, I mean it. Take a deep breath. What happened to your upper body when you did that? If your chest expanded and your shoulders rose, then you aren't breathing properly. Don't be ashamed—most of us don't breathe correctly all the time. What we fail to do is to use our diaphragms to take advantage of more of our lungs' capacity.

You've probably heard of singers, wind instrument musicians, and actors talking about the importance of breathing through the diaphragm. They do it because it helps them to control the amount of air they are using. Using proper breathing technique is important for any activity or just daily living, but it is especially important that you breathe properly when working out.

Consciously using your diaphragm is the most efficient way to breathe. The diaphragm is a large, dome-shaped muscle located at the base of your lungs. Your abdominal muscles help move the diaphragm and give you more power to empty your lungs. When you don't use your diaphragm to breathe properly, air can get trapped in your lungs. That air pushes down on your diaphragm and can flatten the dome shape of the muscle and weaken it. When you don't breathe properly, the neck and muscles have to pitch in and that means the diaphragm is working even less. In breathing properly, think of gathering the last 10 percent of air in your lungs.

Diaphragmatic breathing will help you use your diaphragm correctly while breathing to:

- Strengthen the muscle
- Decrease the work of breathing by slowing your breathing rate
- Decrease oxygen demand
- Use less effort and energy to breathe

Breathing techniques are different in toning than in yoga. You will breathe through your diaphragm in both. While doing the toning exercises you will want to breathe naturally in through the nose and out through the mouth, exhaling on the effort. While doing yoga you will breathe both in and out through your nose.

Here's how to properly breathe through your diaphragm. It's a simple and natural process (if you fall asleep on your back, you can't help but breathe this way) that will soon become second nature to you when you are working out.

1. Lie on your back on a flat surface or in bed, with your knees bent and your head supported. You can use a pillow under your knees to support your legs. Place one hand on your upper chest and the other just below your rib cage. This will allow you to feel your diaphragm move as you breathe.
2. Breathe in slowly through your nose so that your stomach moves out against your hand.
3. Tighten your stomach muscles, letting them fall inward as you exhale through pursed lips. Keep the hand on your upper chest as still as possible.

When you first learn the diaphragmatic breathing technique, it'll be easier for you to follow the instructions lying down. When you get better at it, you can try the technique while sitting in a chair. Repeat the same steps as above. You can also do this while standing and while exercising. Remember, inhale through the nose and exhale through the mouth.

When your two-year-old is tugging at your pants, you're pregnant, and the dog is barking to go outside, you need to take in five deep breaths! It's a good stress reliever, and why you usually correlate yoga with breathing.

You'll also find that this breathing technique will help you relax! If you're having trouble sleeping at night, use this technique to inhale deeply for six seconds and exhale fully for six seconds. In no time at all you should relax enough to drift off to sleep!

GATHER YOUR GEAR

For my pregnancy workout plan you will need a few items. None of them are expensive, and some are household items that you probably already have. What you will need:

- A yoga mat or a beach towel
- Three pillows for third trimester
- Two sets of dumbbell weights: one set between two and five pounds and the other set between six and twelve pounds. I use six and twelve pounds. Veterans, use the ones you've been using; no need to decrease weight if you've been exercising. Beginners should start at the lower end. And don't worry—I choreographed these workouts so you can use the same dumbbells throughout, even though you will have a heavier weight growing!

What Size Weights Should I Use?

According to ACSM, if you perform a repetition and a lack of control is evident, you've done too much or your weight is too heavy.

The final requirement is time. I think it is best to work out at the same time each day, but I know that isn't always possible. Some people like to exercise in the morning, others in the evening or at night. It doesn't matter to me, but please do listen to your body and adjust accordingly. For me, exercise started my day off right, and made me a little less nauseous.

GIVE YOURSELF A BREAK

It's important that you understand that your body will tell you when you need a break—both during the workout itself and on those days when you just don't have the energy to work out. Surprisingly, you will probably feel more energized if you work out than if you skip it, but if your fatigue is serious enough that you just can't drag yourself through the routine, don't do it.

You will need to know the difference between tired and fatigued. The first is usually a mental lack of energy and focus; the second is your body telling you that you just don't have the necessary energy reserves to do the

PREGNANCY INTENSITY SCALE

0	Easy	The feeling you get when sitting
1		Activities such as getting dressed
2		The feeling you might get while doing laundry
3		Taking a casual walk
4		Walking briskly, but still maintaining conversation
5	Medium	The feeling you get when rushing out the door
6		The feeling you get when rushing up a flight of stairs
7		You are able to exercise while singing
8		Slightly tiring exercise, but you're still speaking full sentences
9		Feeling fatigue; breathing hard
10	Maximal	All-out exercise; could not maintain for more than thirty seconds

Please stay between 5 and 8.

work. If you feel light-headed, short of breath, painfully sore, weak in the legs, or some other clear and obvious physical weakness, stop immediately. It is more important for you to figure out why you are feeling that way than it is to get your workout in. One of the likely sources of fatigue is dehydration. Fifty percent of Americans admit to feeling the debilitating effects of dehydration; one of its first effects on the body is fatigue. Consult your journal or review your daily intake if you are feeling fatigue. Another reason for it may be low blood sugar. Again, I can't stress enough the importance of nutritional awareness and how it relates to your whole life, including exercise. You must drink enough and have enough calories in your system to exercise effectively.

Also, you will note that I have scheduled a break for you during your workout. If you need to take additional breaks, do so. As a reminder, on page 77 is the rate of perceived exertion scale that you can use to gauge just how hard you are working. Remember, you should stay between 5 and 8 on the scale.

DON'T CHEAT—COMPETE

I know that it is easy to cheat on this scale and tell yourself that you're working harder than you really are. I also know that it is easy not to do the recommended number of exercises or work for the duration of the activity. One of the reasons why people hire personal trainers is that they need someone to watch over them, to motivate and encourage, and to get on their case when they aren't giving their best effort. So unless you have your own PT coming to work you out, you are going to have to discover your inner PT. Some people are naturally competitive and can push themselves. Some need the encouragement and oversight of others. My rule of thumb is this: Know thyself (and know thy exercise style!). You have to be honest with yourself and know what kind of person you are. If you're not one of those completely self-motivating people, then maybe you need to find a buddy to work out with. For most couples, time together is at a premium, so working out together may be one way to spend a few minutes a day engaged in the same activity. But I know working out with my husband caused a bit of feuding. Telling him to work out every day is like telling me to floss my teeth every day. So we keep our professional opinions to ourselves! I should just bite my tongue and be happy he's working out!

Remember, at the highest level of effort you are expending, you should be able to speak whole sentences without huffing and puffing. Having your partner there will not only motivate you, but by talking together during the workout you will be able to monitor your effort level. Some people find that it is better to work out with a friend instead of a partner, and that's fine too. Just make sure that if you do use a workout buddy, he or she knows what the limits are and what kind of effort you should be putting in. Don't cheat and use a softy as your partner. Get someone who can be firm but fair with you.

Types of Exercise

OK, now that you know some of the basics, we're going to move into the types of exercise that you are going to be doing. Each category of exercise you will be performing has a specific purpose. Here's a brief overview of those types of activities you will be doing and what purpose they serve.

Warm-up: These fairly gentle exercises are designed to get your blood moving through your muscles. The will elevate your heart rate slightly and raise your breathing rate a bit. In terms of the intensity scale, you should be between a 2 and a 4 by the time you complete the first phase. The warm-up is *mandatory* and will remain the same throughout each trimester.

Toning: This is the first component of the main section of the workout. Exercises that tone your body are those that target a specific muscle, muscle group, or area of the body. You will be using weights and doing the lifting while doing other movements; these are called compound, or two-in-one, exercises. Two-in-one exercises raise your heart rate and work multiple muscles. Women are very good at multitasking (this will become even more relevant after the baby gets here), so why shouldn't we multitask the workout? We'll get more done in less time, but I promise it won't be too coordinated. The point here is not to build muscle at all, but to get rid of those fat stores. You will see some definition developing in your muscles, though—they will be outlined more distinctly than before.

Here are a few things to keep in mind about using weights: When you lift the weight, exhale. When you lower the weight, inhale. Repeat after me: Lift out and lower in. Also be sure that you raise and lower the weights slowly and in a controlled manner. You want to keep your muscle activated throughout the movement. That means don't drop them and don't throw them. I don't mean physically releasing them, but don't release the muscles that are working to raise and lower the weights.

Cooldown: In my program, you will always cool down by doing yoga and some easy marching to lower the heart rate slowly. These movements and positions are designed to do the exact opposite of the warm-up. They will allow you to slow your heart rate. I will vary the types of movements you do in each of the trimesters to allow for the changes in your body. It is important that you do the cooldown, since these movements also help rush the flow of blood to your muscles (including your uterus), giving them the nutrients they need to repair cellular-level damage and to flush out any toxins that have been released. If you are sore after exercise, it is because your muscles need to repair this cellular damage and flush toxins. Your body's inflammatory response will kick in. Cooling down limits the damage and often shortcuts the inflammation response.

Working Your Core: If you remember nothing else and do nothing else that I recommend, the core is the single most important element of this program. Your core is essentially the center of your body—more specifically your abdominal muscles, pelvic floor, hips, and back. They are among the largest muscles. And your core work is done after the cooldown, since we want to return your heart rate in a safe manner before you exercise on the floor.

The illustration below shows you the location of the major abdominal

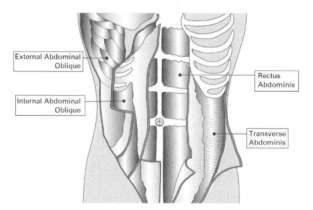

The muscles of the core. There is a layer of fascia that covers your muscles to act as a sheath and keep you compact.

muscles. I'll give you guidance on how to locate those muscles on your own body to make certain that you are engaging them properly while doing the exercises.

Your abdominal wall is divided into four parts. The external obliques are at the top and the outside of your abdomen. The internal obliques run below their counterpart. What we commonly refer to as the "six-pack" is the rectus abdominis, which sits on the top of the stomach and descends along the midline of the body. Finally, the transverse abdominis, or TA, is the deep abdominal muscle that runs under the six-pack. It is the most important of the muscle groups of the abdomen. The pelvic floor (PF) and TA keep your belly from dropping to your toes. The TA and PF, together with the uterus, work to push your baby out during delivery. The stronger they are pre-delivery, the easier your labor should be. And the easier it will be to get your body back!

Fascia covers the muscles and acts as a sheath to keep your waist compact. Of course, if your muscles are not toned underneath there is a lot more compacting for the fascia to do! After birth your fascia will be back to 90 percent of its original strength within six weeks; the other 10 percent will come back within a year. You cannot strengthen or tighten your fascia without surgery, so preventive measures are necessary!

Do you need another reason to stay within your recommended weight gain? Not only will your fascia bounce back quicker, but you can avoid stretch marks in most cases. If you gain weight gradually, and not too much, you can keep stretch marks at bay.

Getting to the Bottom of the Core

Think of the pelvic floor as the bottom of the core, and visualize a sling from front to back. You will start by finding your pelvic floor, then training it. The pelvic floor is the foundation to your core; your abs cannot function without it. It is important for a number of reasons: It helps with incontinence and post-partum issues, and training the pelvic floor can help create the flat stomach you're looking for.

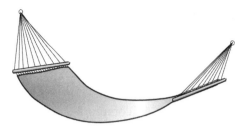

Your pelvic floor is like a hammock, holding up your core.

Together the four muscle groups of the abdominal wall, especially the TA, and the muscles of the pelvic floor act as a sling supporting your baby. Again, the stronger you can get these muscles, the more comfortable you will be before, during, and after delivery. If you want to be able to wiggle into your skinny jeans or wear that bikini without your pooch folding over your swimsuit's bottom, then working your core is essential.

Finding Your Transverse Abdominis and Pelvic Floor

Lie on your back with your feet close to your butt. Pull your hip bones toward your rib cage and perform a Kegel. If you felt your legs or your buttocks tense you were not using your pelvic floor; you were using your lower body muscles. Try it again, this time with your feet up on a chair. If you're able to pull your hip bones down and flatten your belly without engaging your butt or your leg muscles, you've done it! You've hit bottom and used the muscles of your transverse abdominis and pelvic floor.

Kegels are simple exercises you can do to exercise your pelvic floor while sitting, standing, or getting ready for bed. And nobody will even notice you're "exercising." Contract your muscles as though you are stopping the flow of urine, hold for ten seconds, and release. Repeat as often as you like, aiming for several sets throughout the day.

Core 101: An Introduction

Using the transverse abdominis muscle is a big part of my core workout technique. As you can see from the illustration on page 80, the TA is a thick layer of muscle that runs wraps around the torso. The muscle fibers of the TA are your true core muscles, and strengthening them will give you power and tone your entire body. The muscle action is the same during pregnancy; now there is just a baby under your muscles!

> In order to fully engage your abdominals, and in particular your TA muscle, you have to pull your belly button in toward your spine. This engages the TA, and works the other muscles that run along your spine as well as your abdominals. You probably engage these muscles without even knowing it when you put on your skinny jeans.
>
> Pulling your belly button toward your spine is *not* the same thing as sucking in your gut. What do you do when you suck in your gut? You hold your breath. You don't want to do that. When you are lying on your back and you suck in your gut and hold your breath, what else happens? Try it and find out.
>
> That's right. Your chest rises. That's not what you're trying to do. You want the chest to be still when you pull your abdominal muscles toward your spine. When you are lying on your back, think about someone putting a foot on your belly and compressing it down toward the floor. You can still breathe normally (and that's when your chest can rise and fall), but you aren't holding your expanded chest still.

The CFS Method

In Part II, after you've had your baby and are really able to work your core muscles, we will talk about the Core Firing Sequence (CFS) method. Each of the muscles discussed above needs to be worked, and the method that I recommend will allow you to work them all and in the proper order so that you will maximize the benefits of the exercise you are doing.

Healthy muscles are very resilient and can bounce back. Getting rid of that little bit of belly is what most women want to do post-pregnancy, and by following the guidance I provide, you will do so with minimum time and maximum results.

> Diastasis recti is a condition that up to 60 percent of women experience during pregnancy. The word *diastasis* means "separation," and *recti* refers to the rectus abdominis, the center muscle that is your six pack. What happens as a result of your expanding

belly is this muscle can become separated from the linea alba, the line of fibrous tissue that runs down the midline of your abdomen. It separates your rectus abdominis muscles into a left and right side. Sometimes, as your baby develops and your abdomen expands, a slight separation of the muscle from the dividing tissue can occur, resulting in diastasis recti.[32] If you have this condition, then you should not do the core exercises I've outlined for you during your second and third trimesters. Generally, women don't have this separation during the first trimester, but if you experience any discomfort in this area, you may want to ease up on the core exercises.

The condition is not serious and in most cases will heal after the baby is out. Because it is caused by the expanding of your belly, those of you who are carrying twins or who are having a larger baby are more susceptible to it. In Part II, I instruct you on a number of exercises that you can do postpartum to ensure that you heal properly, but for now just remember that doing core exercises will help now and later.

SELF-TESTING FOR DIASTASIS RECTI

Lie on your back with your belly exposed. Bring your feet up toward your butt. Find your belly button, and place the middle finger of one hand an inch above it and pointing toward your feet. Place your pointer and ring fingers against the sides of your middle finger; gently press in. If all three of your fingers sink into a gap between your abdominis recti muscles, then you have diastasis recti. If only one or two fit easily in that gap, then you don't have the condition. In the photo below, you can see the correct position of the fingers. This photo shows the normal state:

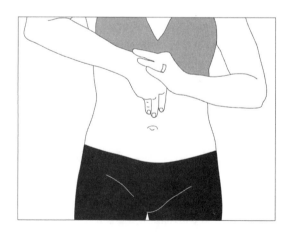

Self-testing for diastasis recti

You can also watch the Moms Into Fitness video at youtube.com/momsintofitness and self-test for diastasis recti both during pregnancy and afterward.

Cardio/Aerobic Workouts

Another major component of your workout during all three trimesters is the cardio workout. *Cardio* is short for *cardiovascular,* and these activities are designed to elevate your heart rate to improve the level of fitness of your heart, lungs, and circulatory system. You will feel cardio benefits in some of the toning exercises—it's like getting the most bang for your buck. I designed the workouts so you can get them done quickly! Some people use the word *aerobic* to describe these kinds of activities. Because so many people have bad associations with the word, I tend to go with the term *cardio* most of the time. One thing you should know about the word *aerobic* is that it simply means "with oxygen." Activities that require you to bring more oxygen into your system in order to complete them are considered aerobic activities. They work your cardiovascular system. Exercises that don't require the same level of oxygen uptake (weight training, bowling, golf) are said to be anaerobic or "without oxygen." That doesn't mean that you need to hold your breath while doing them, but you won't find yourself in oxygen debt as a result of engaging in them. If you are pregnant with twins you should skip the cardio exercise.

Unless you have been running prior to getting pregnant, I don't advise you to run during pregnancy. If you are a runner, then you can substitute a jog or run in the cardio workouts below when you're asked to do a "speed walk." Obviously, then, the main cardio exercise you will be doing during all three trimesters is walking.

If you like to get cardio and toning done inside and all in one workout, use my DVDs! Go to momsintofitness.com/dvds and click on the pregnancy DVDs.

Keep in mind that you should vary the type of cardio workout you do: endurance or interval. Let's take a look at the difference between the two:

PREGNANCY CARDIO ENDURANCE WALK (HILLS ARE GOOD)

Intensity	Time	Speed
3–5	5 minutes	warm-up (gradually walk up to your normal speed)
5–6	1 minute	walk
7–8	1 minute	speed walk
5–6	2 minutes	walk
7–8	2 minutes	speed walk
5–6	3 minutes	walk
7–8	3 minutes	speed walk
5–6	4 minutes	walk
7–8	4 minutes	speed walk
5–6	5 minutes	walk
7–8	5 minutes	speed walk
3–4	5 minutes	cooldown/slow walk

Use the yoga section in your current trimester for stretching.

INTERVAL WALK

Intensity	Time	Speed
3–5	5 minutes	warm-up walk
6–8	3 minutes	speed walk
5	2 minutes	walk
6–8	3 minutes	speed walk
5	2 minutes	walk
6–8	3 minutes	speed walk
5	2 minutes	walk
6–8	3 minutes	speed walk
5	2 minutes	walk
6–8	3 minutes	speed walk
5	2 minutes	walk
3–4	5 minutes	cooldown/slow walk

Use the yoga section in your current trimester for stretching.

As you can see, with the endurance walk, you incrementally increase the duration of the speed-walking portion and build to peak so that at the end of the walk, you are working at the highest level of intensity for the longest span of time. In the interval walk, you alternate between a slower pace and a faster pace at regular intervals after the warm-up. Both of these are excellent ways to get a good cardio workout. (Consider interval cardio a two-in-one exercise—you get more done in less time because you burn more calories while challenging your endurance.) Another difference between the two is that instead of raising your heart rate to a certain level and leaving it there until the cooldown, you are gradually raising your heart and respiration rates in the case of the endurance walk and raising and lowering it incrementally during the interval walk.

Reserve doing steady-pace walking for those days when you're butt is dragging a bit, but remember that you still need to concentrate on getting something out of the workout. Think about striking the ground heel first and then pushing off with your toes, or imagine that you have a pencil pinched between your butt cheeks and you have to clench those muscles to keep it from falling.

The Plan

For each of the three trimesters, your schedule will be the same, but what you do on your exercise days will vary in terms of the core, toning, and yoga exercises you do. Here's what your week will look like:

Monday: Mandatory warm-up, optional cardio block, toning, cardio block, yoga cooldown, core (total workout is about 25–35 minutes for beginners; 35–45 minutes for veterans)
Tuesday: Pregnancy cardio (35–40 minutes)
Wednesday: Mandatory warm-up, optional cardio block, toning, cardio block, yoga cooldown, core (25–35 minutes for beginners; 35–45 minutes for veterans)
Thursday: Rest.
Friday: Mandatory warm-up, optional cardio block, toning, cardio block, yoga cooldown, core (25–35 minutes for beginners; 35–45 minutes for veterans)
Saturday: Family fun exercise. Go for a walk with your husband and/or kids. If you have a child in soccer or another sport, go to the game or practice and walk around the field or court.
Sunday: Rest.

AFTER WORKOUT

Most of us know the importance of warming up before exercise. But what you do after you work out is just as important in preventing injury and speeding recovery. Marching or walking for a few minutes and some simple stretches (or the yoga positions I suggest) are a great way to keep your blood flowing after exercise. Why do you want to keep that good blood flow going? Because that blood flow carries away any cellular debris and other toxins that your body produced while exercising. People get sore from overtaxing their muscles because they don't properly cool down, resulting in a buildup of lactic acid that makes them feel sore.

Your blood pressure rises when you work out, so it's important to lower it gradually. If you stop suddenly, you can feel light-headed and dizzy—not the condition you want to be in when you're pregnant and your balance is already compromised. The same is true of your body temperature. Bring it back to normal gradually.

You burn a lot of calories while working out, and you use up a lot of your stored fluids, so be sure to replenish both your food and water reserves post-exercise. (But at the same time, don't eat the house down!) You'll feel energized instead of sapped of energy if you do all the things I suggest here.

Conclusion

That's it! That is your weekly routine. In the chapters that follow, I'm going to take you step-by-step through each trimester and show you how to do each exercise, let you know how many of each you should do, and fill you in on other issues related to your pregnancy and fitness. Get ready to get fit!

· 5 ·

FIRST TRIMESTER EXERCISE PLAN

Weeks 4–13

Are you psyched? You should be. You're about to begin an exercise program that will make it far easier to get back the body you want post-pregnancy. With your soon-to-be-fit-me outfit safely on display, your goal statements all written out, and your focus on the future firmly in place, it's time to get physical. I've laid out a program for you that will require a minimum of time and will be a great stress release. Just knowing that devoting less than an hour a day to "me time" will make the rest of the pregnancy, labor, and post-pregnancy easier is a wonderful feeling. Knowing that both now and down the line you will be able to experience the benefits of your efforts should be a powerful motivator.

A quick note about how the program is organized: Because you generally won't know that you are pregnant until four to six weeks after conception, I don't include any exercises for weeks one through three. If you want to do pre-pregnancy workouts, use this week plan.

If you are pregnant with twins, you will skip this plan and begin by using the Second Trimester Exercise Plan, starting on page 118. Since you are larger at any given gestational age, your body and babies are at a different stage. I also ask that you get special permission from your doctor to participate in a workout program. You will stop using this program when you are twenty to twenty-four weeks gestation. **If you are pregnant with high-order multiples you should not work out during your pregnancy.**

MATERNITY WORKOUT WEAR

With slim pickins in maternity workout wear, I thought I would share three staple pieces I wore. I lived in my Urban Mom' 3-in-1 yoga pants. I wore them over my belly for the first half of my pregnancies, and once I got bigger I wore them under my belly. I wore them home from the hospital and several weeks after (and they're so soft I still wear them to bed). And I must mention the camo shorts I wore in the springtime! They're super comfy and have a ton of spandex in them, so they stretch. I loved them so much they are now available on my Web site, momsintofitness .com. And my third workout staple piece comes in many different colors: the Gap maternity rib-knit tanks (once you know your size, it's easiest to buy them on the Web).

Of course, you can Google "maternity fitness wear." The prices at online retailers are a bit higher. But a few staple pieces can take you a long way. And many pieces are combination loungewear and workout wear, so you can continue to wear them throughout the day (always change your undergarments, though).

I continued to wear the same-size sports bra. But many women get larger chests; I just wasn't so lucky! So invest in a few larger sports bras. Some women may even need to wear two at a time for extra support.

And be careful picking your supportive shoes. Your feet can swell and even grow during pregnancy! You may want to buy a pair a half size to one size up. Make sure they are super comfy and supportive (you will be carrying around some extra weight, so your knees and hips need that additional cushion). If you are a runner, I recommend going to the Running Store and having them fit you for a shoe. Also, you may want to invest in two pairs of shoes to keep the foot support going for the whole nine months.

Pre-Workout Activities

1. Hydrate and fuel: Drink and eat.
2. Take ten cleansing diaphragmatic breaths: Inhale and exhale through your nose.
3. Clear your mind: Forget your to-do list for now and take some time for yourself.

Go Green

Instead of buying bottles of water, carry one twenty-four-ounce jug of water with you throughout the day. Drink two to three jugs and wash it at the end of the day.

Exercise Glossary

Because some of you haven't worked out before, you may not be familiar with some of the terms used in the exercise descriptions. The list of terms and their definitions below should be helpful for you as you grow accustomed to the new language of exercise:

Abduction: A motion that moves a body part away from the body's centerline.
Adduction: A motion that brings a body part toward the body's centerline.
Bend: Move around a joint at an angle anywhere from fifteen to ninety degrees.
Flex: Slightly move around a joint at an angle anywhere from one to fourteen degrees.
Neutral head: The orientation point is your chin. Don't raise it or lower it but keep it in direct alignment on the horizontal or vertical axis.
Neutral spine: Keep your spine straight and in direct alignment from your neck to your tailbone. Don't allow it to arch (curve backward so that your head is behind your butt) or hunch (so that your head is in front of your pelvis).
Repetition: The completion of one individual set of actions that make up an exercise.
Set: A predetermined number of repetitions that you expect to complete.
Soft knees: Keep your knees slightly flexed at all times. Don't lock them in position.

Monday, Wednesday, Friday (Weeks 4–13)

Reminders during your workout:

1. Core activation: Keep a neutral spine and keep the abdominals activated by saying the words *ha-ha-ha*. I learned this exercise through the American Council on Exercise, and it's a wonderful reminder to keep the core activated while prego. You will do the same when you are not pregnant—the muscle action is the same, but now there is a baby under those muscles!
2. Perform Kegels: Doing Kegels will help maintain a strong pelvic floor. Contract your muscles as if you are cutting off the flow of urine. Hold this contraction for 10 seconds. Repeat. Remember not to contract the abs, buttocks, or thigh muscles.
3. Take a break when needed.
4. Beginners will do 1 set of 15 of each toning exercise. Veterans will do 2 sets of 15 of each toning exercise with about a 20-second rest between sets.
5. Get your doctor's permission first and *do not* use this book if you are carrying more than two babies.

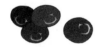

At seven weeks your baby is the size of a blueberry. Blueberries are beneficial to Mom as they are low in calories, contain fiber, and give you vitamins C, B_1, B_2, B_6, and E.

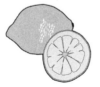

At fourteen weeks your baby is the size of a lemon. Lemons can help you battle nausea, but DO NOT eat them whole!

Mandatory Warm-up (5 minutes)

Minute 1: Step knee

Target: Raise your heart rate and increase blood flow to your muscles.

Start: Stand with your feet shoulder-width apart.

Motion: Bend your arms at the elbows so your forearms are parallel to the floor, and make soft fists. Simultaneously lift your right knee and your left arm. Switch and repeat.

Pointers: Quickly raise your legs and arms to increase the effort and to raise your heart rate. Stay light on your feet; as you touch down with one foot, immediately raise the other.

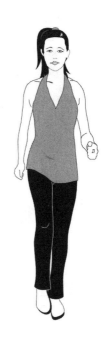

Step knee

Minute 2: Knee pushes

Target: Raise your heart rate and increase blood flow to your muscles.
Start: Stand with your feet shoulder-width apart.
Motion: Bend your arms at the elbows so your forearms are parallel to the floor,
and make soft fists. Simultaneously lift your right knee and both arms. As you
lower your right knee, lower your elbows to your sides and open your hands
so that your palms are facing the ceiling. As you raise your left knee, bring
both of your arms above your head with your palms still facing the ceiling.
Pointers: Quickly raise your legs and arms to raise your heart rate. Stay light on
your feet; as you touch down with one foot, raise the other. Keep your palms
up and your shoulders relaxed. Don't scrunch your neck and shoulder muscles.

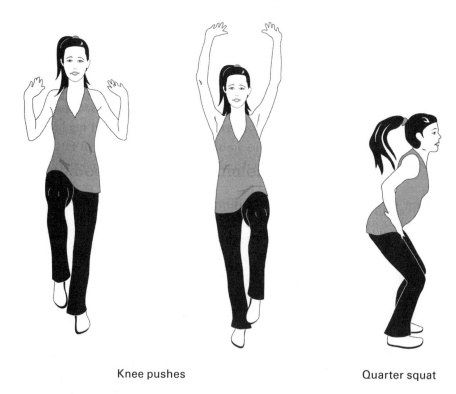

Knee pushes   Quarter squat

Minute 3: Quarter squat

Target: Raise your heart rate and increase blood flow to your muscles.
Start: Place your feet shoulder-width (or farther) apart. Put your hands on
your hips.

Motion: Inhale as you raise your chin; focus your eyes on a point on the ceiling just ahead of you. Bend your hips and your knees as you lower your butt toward the floor. The lowest you should descend is forty-five degrees. Exhale as you return to the starting position.

Pointers: Keep your hands on your hips throughout the exercise. Keep your knees soft and focus on your breathing. Don't drop your chin or lower your eyes! These should be done quickly; shoot for 20–22 reps.

Minute four: Quarter squat and pull

Target: Raise your heart rate and increase blood flow to your muscles.

Start: Place your feet shoulder-width (or farther) apart.

Motion: Inhale as you raise your arms overhead. Perform a quarter squat. As you squat, pull your elbows toward your hips. Then extend your arms above your head as you stand up.

Pointers: Keep your knees soft and focus on your breathing. Don't drop your chin or lower your eyes!

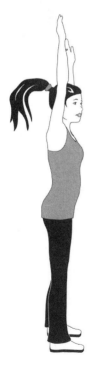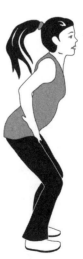

Quarter squat and pull

Minute 5: Alternating side lunge

Target: Raise your heart rate and increase blood flow to your muscles.

Start: Stand with your toes pointing forward and your feet at least shoulder-width apart.

Motion: Place your hands on your hips. Inhale and, with your knees soft, shift your weight to the right. Your left leg should remain straight and your left foot should stay in full contact with the floor. Exhale and shift your weight back to center. Pause for a count of two before shifting your weight to the left.

Pointers: As you shift from center, be sure to bend the knee that will be supporting your weight. You should feel a mild stretch in your inner thighs.

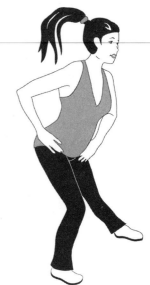

Alternating side lunge

Cardio Block: Optional

See page 104.

Toning Section (12–22 minutes)

If you are a beginner, you will take twelve minutes to finish one set of each exercise. Veterans will take twenty-two minutes to finish two sets of each exercise. While these are suggested times, please exercise at your own pace! Veterans, you have an option of doing two sets with a 20-second rest between or doing 1 set completing the toning portion, then repeat.

Triceps push-up (use stair for modified version)

Target: Triceps (back of arms), deltoids (shoulders), upper back, chest, core (abs, middle-low back).

Start: Begin in the prone (facedown) position. Place your wrists directly under your shoulders so that your body forms a straight line from the top of the head to the knees. Straighten your elbows and lift your body off of the floor, knees down.

Motion: Flex your elbows and extend. Your elbows should remain parallel to your rib cage as you press your weight up.

Pointers: Pull your abs in so there is no arch in the upper body. Try not to let your elbows bow out, which works different muscle groups.

Repetitions: 1 set of 15 for beginners; 2 sets of 15 for veterans

Modification: Place your hands on a stair or other elevated surface if you don't have stairs.

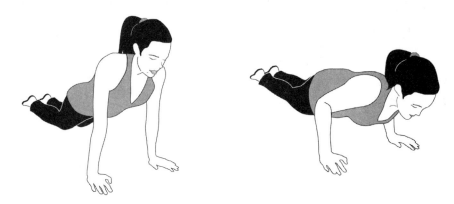

Triceps push-up

Incline chest fly (incline is optional during your first trimester), heavy weights

Target: Chest, back of legs (hamstrings), butt, core (abs, pelvic floor, hips, back).

Start: You will need your heavy weights. Lie in the supine position (on your back) with your knees bent and heels twelve to eighteen inches from your butt. Bend your elbows slightly so they are in line with your shoulders. Your palms should face each other.

Motion: Extend your arms and bring your hands together directly above your midline. Squeeze your chest muscles; extend and release your arms.

Pointers: Emphasize the chest squeeze—imagine you are pressing a ball between your breasts. Don't lock your elbows.

Modification: Elevate your upper body with three pillows or an exercise ball. Start in the incline position with your knees bent.

Warning: Do not use an exercise ball for this exercise if you're pregnant and you have never used one before. Your balance is off during pregnancy, and a ball will increase the likelihood that you will fall over.

Repetitions: 1 set of 15 for beginners; 2 sets of 15 for veterans

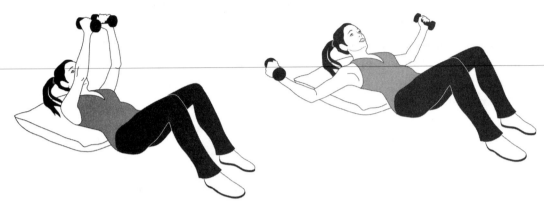

Incline chest fly

Squat to knee, one heavy weight

Target: Quadriceps (front of thighs), hamstrings (back of thighs), glutes (butt), abductors (outer thighs), adductors (inner thighs), calves, core.

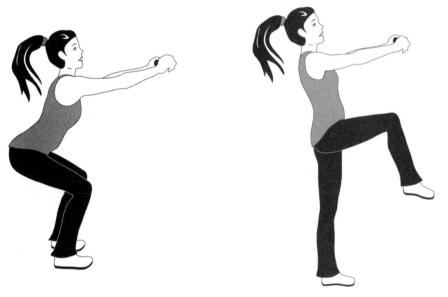

Squat to knee

Start: Stand with your feet shoulder-width (or slightly farther) apart. With your arms straight out in front of you, hold one heavy weight at shoulder height with both hands.

Motion: Flex your hips slightly and then bend your knees to ninety degrees. Keep your knees behind your toes. With your knees flexed, in one fluid motion sit into the squat. As you come back up, exhale and raise your right leg, keeping your knee bent. Maintain a neutral spine. Alternate lifting legs.

Pointers: Extend through the supporting leg. Keep your knees behind your toes in the squat.

Modification: Use a light weight or no weight.

Repetitions: 1 set of 15 for beginners; 2 sets of 15 for veterans

Squeeze and press, light weights

Target: Deltoids (shoulders), triceps (backs of arms), core (abs, back, pelvic floor, hips).

Start: Place your elbows next to your body at a ninety-degree angle with a weight in each hand. Your palms should face each other.

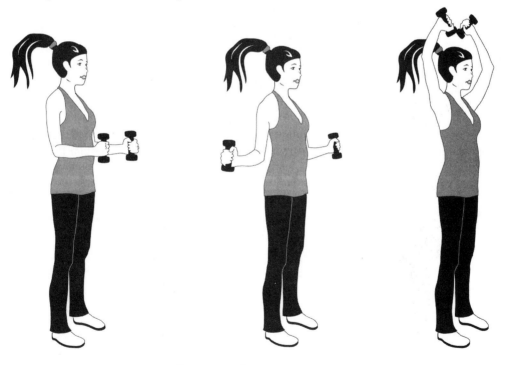

Squeeze and press

Motion: With your elbows against your sides, bring your hands away from your body. Keep your elbows at a 90-degree angle as you press your arms overhead. Return your elbows to your hips, and bring your palms back to each other.

Pointers: Engage your abdominals. The only part of your body that moves is your arms. Keep your core straight.

Modification: Sit in a chair if you can't maintain a neutral spine.

Repetitions: 1 set of 15 for beginners; 2 sets of 15 for veterans

Reverse lunge and curl, heavy weights

Target: Quadriceps (front of thighs), hamstrings (back of thighs), glutes (buncakes), abductors (outer thighs), adductors (inner thighs), calves, biceps.

Start: With weights in your hands and arms extended, bring your elbows to the sides of your body, your palms facing outward.

Motion: Step back two to three feet with your right leg. Bend both of your knees to ninety degrees and slightly flex your hips. Keep the majority of your weight on your left foot while keeping your left knee directly over your heel. Simultaneously perform a posture curl by flexing your elbows. Then extend both knees and hips to the upright position, and extend your elbows. Perform one set on your right leg lunge with posture curls, then switch to your left leg lunge without posture curls.

> The reason you do posture curls as opposed to biceps curls is to open your chest as you gain weight in your belly. If you have carpal tunnel you need to perform regular biceps curls.

Pointers: Keep your front knee directly over your ankle. Push through your front heel. Try not to lift your elbows from your sides.

Repetitions: 1 set of 15 for beginners; 2 sets of 15 for veterans

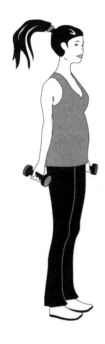 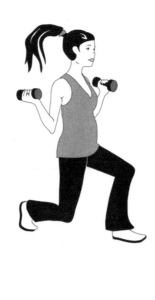

Reverse lunge and curl

Break and hydrate.

Drink water!

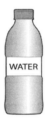

WATER

Quadruped triceps kickback, one light weight

Target: Triceps (back of arms), rear deltoids (back of shoulders), core.
Start: Kneel on all fours. Align your hips directly above your knees and your shoulders directly above your hands. Keep your head aligned with your spine. Flex your right arm to ninety degrees with a weight in your hand. Elevate your right elbow above your hips with your palm facing forward.
Motion: Fully extend your arm, keeping your elbow stationary. Return your arm to ninety degrees. Perform 1 set on the right, then 1 set on the left.

Pointers: For a more intense workout, raise your elbow higher. Keep your wrist straight as you bring the weight back.

Modification: If the wrist of your supporting arm hurts, place your other weight on the floor, wrap your hand around it, and keep your wrist straight.

Repetitions: 1 set of 15 for beginners; 2 sets of 15 for veterans

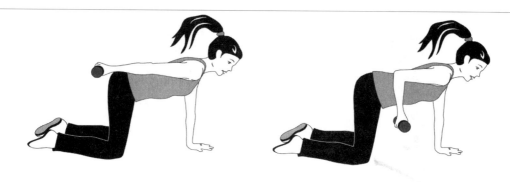

Quadruped triceps kickback

Curtsy to abduct, heavy weights

Target: Adductors (inner thighs), abductors (outer thighs), glutes (butt), core.

Start: Stand with your feet shoulder-width apart. Hold weights in each hand. Shift your weight onto your right leg, with your left foot a few inches off the floor.

Motion: Extend your left leg one to two feet behind you diagonally and to the right, with your heel lifted. Bend your knees to a ninety-degree angle. Return to starting position and extend your left leg out to the side. Perform all of your reps on your right side before switching to the left side.

Pointers: Bend both knees and keep your front heel on the floor. Do not let your knees extend past your toes when you bend down. Keep the knee of the abducting leg forward, not up.

Modification: Do not extend your non-supporting leg; instead return to starting position before performing the next rep.

Repetitions: 1 set of 15 for beginners; 2 sets of 15 for veterans

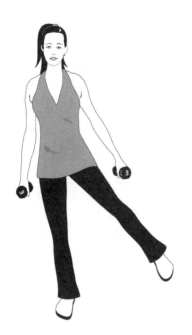

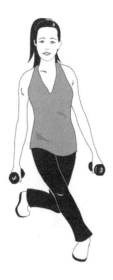

Curtsy to abduct

Plié and pull, light weights

Target: Abductors (outer thighs), adductors (inner thighs), quadriceps (front of legs), hamstrings (back of legs), glutes (butt), core, triceps (back of arms), deltoids (shoulders).

Start: Stand with your legs wider than shoulder width and your toes pointed out forty-five degrees or more. With a weight in each hand, extend your arms above your head.

Motion: Lower yourself, bending your knees and hips. Ideally, you should be able to get your hips level with your knees. At the same time, lower the weights to shoulder level by bending your elbows and pulling down toward the middle of your back. Return to the starting position. Keep a neutral spine throughout.

Pointers: Keep your weight on your heels. Do not let your knees go past your toes when lowering yourself. Don't arch your back or bend forward! Keep your spine neutral.

Repetitions: 1 set of 15 for beginners; 2 sets of 15 for veterans

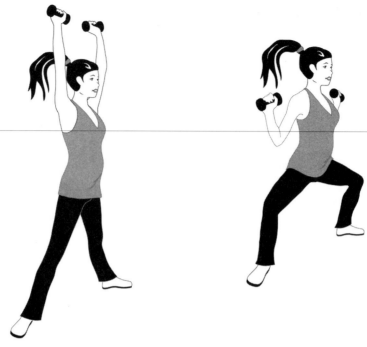

Plié and pull

Cardio Block

Perform each of the following for thirty to forty-five seconds, taking a break in between exercises if necessary.

1. **Prego jacks:** Jump out to quarter squat and jump in.
2. **Mini-rope:** Pretend jump-rope.
3. **Lateral ski:** Hop sideways from one leg to the other.

Yoga Breathing

In yoga, practitioners use many different breathing techniques. For our purposes, we're going to simplify things a bit and state that while doing these poses, you should use the diaphragmatic breathing technique discussed earlier. Remember that you are trying to fill your belly with air as if it were a balloon. Inhale and exhale through your nose. Each breath should last a count of twelve—six on the inhale and six on the exhale.

4. Push knees: Just like the warm-up but faster.
5. Stairs or knees, like in the warm-up.

Yoga Cooldown (8–10 Minutes)

3-minute march-in-place cooldown (march slowly; you should be bringing your heart rate down)

NOTE: You will hold each pose through five deep yoga breaths. Do not close your eyes since you are pregnant.

Bow and arrow

- Stand and place your feet wide apart.
- Make sure the heels of both feet are in a straight line. Your torso should be straight and facing forward.
- Flex your knees and lean to the left so that 70 percent of your weight is on your left leg. Your left knee should block your left foot from view if you were to look down.
- Extend your left arm above your head.
- With your right hand grab the outside of your right ankle and bring your heel toward your butt.
- Do diaphragmatic breathing while holding this posture and gazing steadily a few feet in front of you.
- With every breath, engage your mind, and feel yourself expanding and growing more and more powerful. Keep your gaze steadily focused, with the intent of breaking through all obstacles and barriers.
- After five deep yoga breaths reverse the direction of the posture by coming out of it the way you went in.
- To modify, follow the first illustration and do not perform the exercise in the second illustration.
- Repeat on your other side.

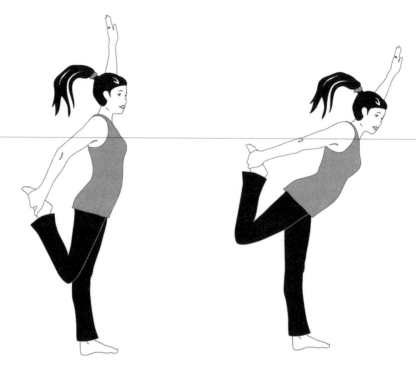

Bow and arrow

WARRIOR TO PYRAMID

Hold each pose for five breaths.

Warrior II

- Begin with your feet shoulder-width apart and your arms out to the sides at shoulder level, parallel to the floor.
- Widen your stance until your legs are three and a half to four feet apart.
- Keep your back straight, tailbone down, and pelvis lifted but not tilted forward.
- Turn your right foot ninety degrees out and your left foot approximately forty-five degrees inward. The arch of your left foot should be aligned with the heel of your right foot.
- As you exhale, slowly turn your torso toward your right leg.

- Keep your left leg strong as you bend your right leg into a ninety-degree angle, knee over the ankle.
- Gaze past your front fingers.

Warrior I

- From Warrior II raise your arms parallel above your head, palms facing in. Reach them actively upward, arms tight, shoulders down.

Pyramid

- From Warrior I lower your hands to your right shin or upper thigh (whichever your flexibility allows).
- Simultaneously straighten your right leg with a slight bend at the knee.

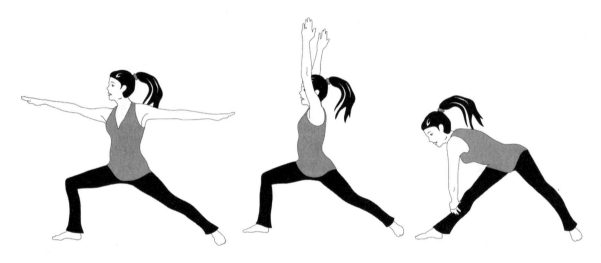

Warrior to pyramid

Windshield wiper

- Place your hands on your hips with your feet hip-width apart and knees slightly bent.
- Step back, then hinge at your hips as you sit back, placing the majority of your weight on your back leg.

- Straighten your front leg, flexing your foot toward you.
- With your front foot, perform a motion like a slow windshield wiper. Repeat five times with one breath each rep.
- Advanced modification: Feel a deeper stretch in your hips by keeping the same position as above, but move your hips side to side like a windshield wiper.
- Beginner modification: Place your hands on a wall in front of you instead of on your hips.
- Repeat other side.

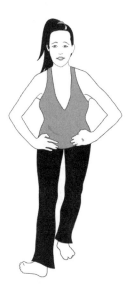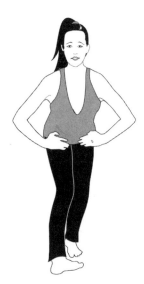

Windshield wiper

Half moon to supported arch

- Stand with your feet together.
- Inhale as you lift your right arm overhead; exhale and lean to your left with your left hand on your hip. Hold here as you inhale and exhale five times. Then repeat on the other side.
- Advanced modification: Come out of this position into a supported arch. Place both hands on the small of your back, fingers pointing down. Inhale and exhale as you slightly arch your back.

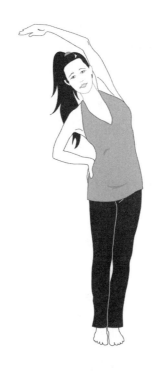

Half moon to
supported arch

Squat pose

- Stand with your feet two to three feet apart, toes pointed out forty-five degrees or more.
- Slowly bend your knees, keeping your spine tall, and glide your hands along your thighs as you sit into a deep squat.
- Your goal is to reach your hands toward the floor while keeping your head above your heart. Hold for five deep breaths.
- Beginner modification: If you cannot get this deep into the squat, face a wall and glide your hands down along the wall until you are comfortable.

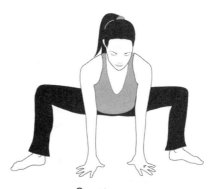

Squat pose

Reclined fold

- Lie on your back. Optional: Lie on an incline (two or three pillows under your upper body).

- Grab your calves (or the back of your knees) with your hands.
- Inhale, then exhale, pulling your straight legs toward your body. Repeat for five breaths.
- Beginner modification: Grab behind your knees. Inhale, then exhale, pulling your knees toward your body as you keep your legs bent.

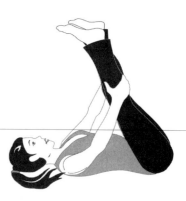

Reclined fold

Downward dog to child's pose

- Lower yourself to the floor so that you're on your hands and knees with wrists beneath your shoulders and knees below your hips.
- Curl your toes under and push yourself back with your arms while raising your hips and straightening your legs.
- Keeping your hands in place, rotate your upper arms outward to widen your collarbones and expand your chest.
- Let your head hang. Prevent yourself from scrunching your shoulders around your ears by moving your shoulder blades away and toward your hips.
- Engage your quadriceps to take the weight off your arms, making this a resting pose.
- As a beginner, you may not be able to bring your heels down flat; your muscles may still be too tight to accomplish this. Resist the temptation to walk your hands back toward your feet to help bring your heels all the way down. Cheating like this won't help lengthen the muscles. Eventually you will be able to achieve the heels-flat position. Be patient. It will take some time for all the muscles to lengthen.
- Transition to child's pose: Bring your knees to the mat, then sit back on your feet with your knees wide.
- Slowly bend forward until you can rest your forehead on the floor directly in front of you. Keep your arms forward, resting on the floor.

- Settle into a comfortable position by wiggling.
- Focus on your breathing and relaxing all your muscles.
- Hold for five breaths.
- If you can't get comfortable in this position, fold your arms in front of you and rest your head on them.

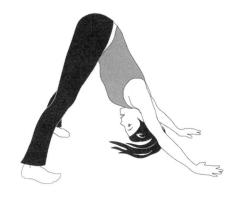

Downward dog

Core Workout (3–5 minutes)

Lindsay's reminder: Continue performing the ha-ha-ha until it becomes a habit.

Four-count transverse crunch: Kegel, pelvic tilt, transverse, crunch (cough up).

Start: Lie in the supine position with your knees bent and your heels close to your butt.

Motion: Keep your lower back on the floor while you engage your abs and raise your chest and shoulders six inches off the floor. Your elbows should be bent and your interlocked hands should support your head. 1) Perform a Kegel (see pages 123–124 for a description) and hold the contraction. 2) Pull your hip bones toward your rib cage and perform a pelvic tilt without squeezing your buttocks. 3) Pull your belly button down toward your spine, look at your belly button, and 4) crunch or "cough up." After the crunch, lower yourself so that your shoulder blades graze the floor. Repeat steps 1 through 4.

Pointers: Exhale on the exertion and inhale on the rest. Don't use your arms to pull yourself up—just support your head; don't lift it with your arms.

Repetitions: 1 set of 15 for beginners; 1 set of 25 for veterans

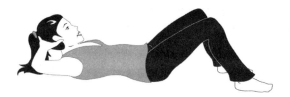

Four-count transverse crunch

Plank abductions

Start: Lying facedown on the floor, place your palms on the floor directly under your shoulders. Keep your arms and legs straight as you do a push-up. Pull your navel in so your body forms a straight line from the top of your head to your toes. Try not to let your hips flex. Push the floor away to fully support your upper body. Hold this position.

Motion: Slightly raise one leg and abduct (move it away from your midline), then return to center. Repeat with your other leg. Alternate leg abductions.

Pointers: Try to maintain a straight head-to-toe alignment. Imagine wires connected to the top of your head and the soles of your feet pulling you in opposite directions.

Modification: Hold plank position, resting both kness on the ground.

Repetitions: 2 × 30 seconds with 20-second rest between

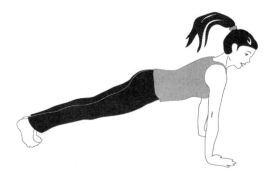

Plank abduction

Double knees or rowboats (beginners do double knees; veterans do rowboats)

Start: Lean back on an incline with your elbows below your shoulders. For rowboats, lean back on an incline with your hands below your shoulders.

Motion: Draw your upper back muscles together and bend your knees so that your heels are close to your body. Pull your knees toward your chest and lift your toes about six inches off the floor. Return to starting position. For rowboats, extend your legs, then pull your knees toward your chest.

Modification: Modify by lifting one leg at a time. For rowboats, modify by doing double knees.

Repetitions: 1 set of 15 for beginners and veterans

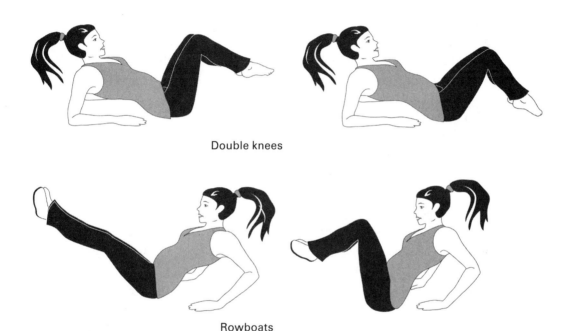

Double knees

Rowboats

Tuesday (Weeks 4–13)

PREGNANCY CARDIO ENDURANCE WALK (HILLS ARE GOOD)

Refer to page 86. Use the scale on page 14 to gauge your walking intensity. Note: As you progress in your pregnancy it will take less work to get to your 7–8 on the intensity scale. Therefore your cardio walk may be less intense in your second and third trimesters.

OR

POST-WORKOUT

Doing the child's pose at the end of your yoga cooldown is a great way to conclude your session. Cooling down is just as important—maybe even more important—as warming up. It is essential, but so is what you do in the hours after your workout is over. How you treat yourself post-workout will go a long way toward determining how sore you will or won't be, how capable your muscles will be of repairing cellular damage and building new and more abundant muscle fibers, and whether or not you have enough fluids in your system to take that good energy with you.

Your cooldown will allow your heart rate to return to its resting state slowly and steadily. If you just stop without the cooldown, you could feel dizzy or even pass out because of the major fluctuation in your blood pressure.

Stretching muscles is a subject of wide debate in the fitness community. You hear all kinds of things about whether or not you should stretch before you warm up (a bad idea, I think, because your muscles are cold and tight), after you warm up, after you get to the heart of your workout, or after the workout.

My belief is this: Gentle stretching after you work out is the best approach to take. And I mean gentle. When you are pregnant your connective tissues are less pliable than they are pre-pregnancy. As a result, it would be easier to strain or more seriously damage a tendon, ligament, etc. Stretching helps to flush out cellular waste products, which are what makes you sore.

It is just as important to hydrate after you exercise as it is to hydrate before. You should drink two to three cups (eight to sixteen ounces) of water within two hours of finishing your workout. In my mind, that's the minimum amount. And keep drinking after that. As with stretching, the water will help flush your system and your baby's. One thing stretching can't do is help your baby's kidney and liver function, but drinking water can.

Finally, you burn calories while working out, so you need to replenish them. Post-workout is a good time to get complex carbohydrates. These are among the foods that your body can metabolize (turn into energy) quickly and steadily. If you can, add some protein. I'm a big believer in the apple-and-peanut-butter snack. You get complex carbs, fiber, protein, and some good fat.

Refer to page 86. Use the scale on page 14 to gauge your walking intensity.

Runners

If you have been jogging, you can do it as long as you feel comfortable. Please replace the speed walks with jogging.

Pregnancy Walking Tips

- Carry a water bottle with you to avoid dehydration, which can cause premature contractions and possibly raise body temperature to a dangerous degree.
- Your gait, or how you walk, is changing to account for extra weight. Pay attention to posture so you don't hurt your back.
- Keep your head straight, your chin level, your hips tucked under the shoulders to avoid swaying, and your eyes focused in front of you. (This is no time to be tripping.)
- Swing your arms to aid balance and intensify the workout.

Exercising Through Morning Sickness or Fatigue

You're not going to feel good every day of this or any of your trimesters, but the first trimester is perhaps the most trying of all. This is the time when your body is undergoing its most radical changes and it hasn't had the time to adapt. Your brain and your attitude haven't had a chance to adapt either. As a result, the twin demons of morning sickness and fatigue may try to lure you back into bed or onto the couch so that you can skip a day. Here are some tips to help you resist:

- Make rest and relaxation a priority.
- Cut back on chores or unnecessary things, or have somebody help you.
- Get extra sleep at night or take a short nap during the day; your body is telling you something.

- Eat well-balanced meals.
- Remember, too much rest and not enough exercise can make morning sickness and fatigue worse!
- Divide your exercise into two or three sessions throughout the day.
- You should feel exhilarated, not drained, after the exercise.
- As you begin to feel better, gradually increase the level of activity.

MAKING HEALTH A HABIT

- Try to eat at least 80 percent of your calories from healthy foods, and the remaining 20 percent from what you want.
- Stock up on portable, healthy snacks for those on-the-go moments.
- Cook double batches of dinner for quick lunches.
- Drink water throughout the day and eliminate soda.
- Get enough sleep.
- Use frozen veggies or prepackaged fresh veggies in a steam bag (my favorite is steamed with some cheddar sprinkles or olive oil and salt and pepper); they are packaged at their ripest and it is easy to steam healthy frozen dinners or ready-to-cook meals instead of eating fast food.
- Take as many steps as you can throughout the day, inside and outside.
- No BLTs (bites, licks, or tastes).
- And, of course, try to fit in some form of exercise at least five times a week.

A Good Start

I once heard the expression "How you start is how you finish." That means that getting off on the right foot, or putting your best forward, is important. Some people say that you only have one chance to make a good first impression. Well, that means almost the same thing, but how to interpret it is like this: If you get off to a good start in developing the proper habits of nutrition and fitness during your first trimester, then you've gone a long way toward setting up a path of success that will lead you from your first pre-pregnancy workout through the lifestyle phase long after you've given birth.

I know that I'm treading on touchy ground here. I also believe that it is never too late to start, that even if you didn't exercise during your first two pregnancies, all you have to do is *start*. What I'm offering here is the best-case scenario. When it comes to exercise, the only worst-case scenario is to not do it at all. So if you're reading this after having gone through your first workout, then you need to stop for a minute and give yourself a round of applause.

· 6 ·

SECOND TRIMESTER EXERCISE PLAN

Weeks 14–27

Pregnant with twins? You will begin your pregnancy workouts with the second trimester exercise plan. For weeks four through thirteen, you will skip the cardio block and all cardio workouts. I also ask that you skip the core section. ACOG suggests that women carrying multiples should refrain from aerobic exercise, so I have adjusted the workout for you. But, again, do what your doctor says is best, which could be swimming or prenatal yoga *only*.

You're doing a good job of strengthening your core muscles and your pelvic floor so that you can better support your rapidly developing baby and ensure that you will have as smooth a delivery as possible. At this point, exercise should feel like a part of your regular routine and is something that you look forward to doing each day. But I know for some of you it's like cleaning the house—you don't want to do it but you know you have to.

If all is going well, you feel a little bit better than you did your first trimester. Exercise should be giving you more energy, helping you to sleep better, and reducing your stress level. That's a win-win for you, your baby, your partner, and everyone else you come into contact with. If you ask my husband it was always more of a win-win for him, because he heard less complaining and heard fewer chunks hitting the toilet. But life is still filled with potential sources of stress, whether or not you're pregnant. Here's a list of things you can do to help ease the potential tension.

Five Ways to Relax

We hear it whether we are pregnant or caring for four children: "Just relax," or "Take a nap." Obviously much easier said than done. Provided below are some mom-approved ways to ease stress, or ways to relax.

- Take a walk.
- Clean for fifteen minutes if you are unable to de-stress while looking at the mess.
- Drink hot tea.
- Play with your kids.
- Call a friend, or your mom.

I hope you can include this book in your list of favorites, and that you find it useful in working up a sweat. While I can't offer you a hot cup of tea, you can count on me as someone who understands what you've been dealing with and can assure you that the results are worth the effort.

A good friend of mine shared with me this tip about keeping her house as neat and orderly as possible; she called it the "one-minute rule": It will take less than one minute to put the lunch dishes in the dishwasher, wipe off the bathroom sink, or put the laundry in the washer—so do it! That's a lot less time than you'll spend being agitated by what a mess you think things are. You'll find your day is much less stressful and your to-do list is a lot smaller if you do small things throughout the day. One task you shouldn't take on is cleaning out your cat's litter box. The chemicals contained in the litter (and the fecal matter in the litter!) are not good for you, so you should consider not having to do this one unpleasant task a blessing.

I know that one potential source of stress is the number of questions you have running through your head. In the spirit of learning some new truths and dispelling some myths, I went to my favorite OB, Dr. Kent Snowden, for these answers, but you should *always* consult with your physician.

1. When will I be released to exercise?
   - If you had a vaginal delivery and no stitches, three to four weeks.
   - If you had a C-section or any stitches from a vaginal delivery, six weeks minimum.

- Six weeks from birth, the fascia of all patients (except those who had multiple births) will be at about 90 percent of its eventual strength; the other 10 percent can take up to a year to get back. The fascia is what keeps your abdomen compact, and is considered the strong part of the abdomen.
- If you were to exercise before being released by your doctor, you could pop a stitch or cause a hernia. But Kegels and pelvic floor work are OK—consult with your physician.

The transition is slow. Take it easy until you feel good!

2. Do C-section patients have a harder recovery than vaginal births regarding physical activity? Or is it just a longer road to recovery?
   - Yes, it's a longer road to recovery; it's like having a cast on your arm.

3. Does a C-section cut through your abdominal muscles?
   - A transverse C-section does not. (See page 176.)

4. In a "normal" delivery, how long before a woman can expect to get her body back?
   - That depends on how much weight a patient gains during pregnancy, her lifestyle, and her exercise habits.

5. Is breast-feeding recommended as a weight-loss trick?
   - Most patients will lose weight doing it.

6. Is it a fact or a myth that once you have three periods your body will let go of the excess fat?
   - Myth!

7. Should I stop exercising as I get close to delivery?
   - If you are pregnant with a singleton, use common sense and stop exercising if you are not feeling well.
   - If you are working out too hard, you can divert the blood flow from the placenta and uterus.
   - If you have any problems or contractions, *stop*. Don't go to exhaustion or get overheated. Otherwise, do what feels good.

8. I am pregnant with twins. Should I exercise?
   - Sure, but after twenty-four to twenty-six weeks take it easy. And consult with your physician.

Take time to eat, drink (not alcohol), and relax throughout the day.

Pregnancy and Stress

As you know from the previous chapter, before you work out, I ask that you clear your mind. With all the questions you have and all the responsibilities you've got, how do you go about clearing your mind when it's hard enough clearing the breakfast dishes? Working out is supposed to help you to de-stress, but it won't work if you aren't able to get in the right frame of mind to begin with. Reducing stress is important for everyone, but particularly for pregnant women—I don't want to stress you by saying this, but it is important.

The Fetal and Neonatal Stress Research Group reported that anxiety and stress can have a negative impact on your developing baby and could have some long-term effects such as hyperactivity. I don't know if it's true that people are generally more stressed today than ever before, but the hyperactivity rates in kids are certainly higher. Along with your physical health, it is obviously important to look out for your mental and emotional health. Meditation and relaxation techniques will multiply the positive effects of your exercise routine while also making the delivery process easier.

MEDITATION

Believe it or not, you are already meditating if you are following my program. Concentrating on your breathing is probably the easiest form of meditation you can do. By focusing on breathing in and out through your nose, filling your belly with air, and using your diaphragm, you are meditating. To enhance the effect, you can also pick a point of focus other than your breath. For example, by placing your hand on your belly, you can feel it rise and fall as you inhale and exhale. Meditation doesn't always mean concentrating on something. It can also mean emptying your mind. Before you exercise, or at any other time during the day, you can go off to a quiet place in your house, your yard, or somewhere else out in nature. Make sure you are somewhere you won't be interrupted by anyone else. Close your eyes and let your mind drift. The key here is to not really focus on those thoughts at all. Just let them come in and go right out.

RELAXATION TECHNIQUES

Along with exercising, you can do other very simple things in order to relax. Other forms of exercise such as tai chi, stretching, and yoga are great relaxation modes.

Listening to soothing music also helps a great deal. A lot of New Age instrumental music is effective, and a quick search for relaxation music will produce hundreds of results. I also find that simply being outside in the fresh air and sunshine relaxes me a lot. For people who work in an office, it's easy to fall into the bad habit of staying indoors except to go from the car to the office and then from the office to the car. This is *not good*! Even a few minutes of fresh air is far better than none!

A Quote for Moms to Live By

It's a quote that I live by and have to remind myself of daily: "You cannot solve a problem by worrying about it."

Additional Considerations During Your Second Trimester

CARPAL TUNNEL SYNDROME

Many women develop carpal tunnel syndrome during pregnancy. You will know if you have this condition because you will usually experience a numb or tingling feeling in your thumb, index, and middle fingers. The reason it's somewhat common in pregnancy is the swelling some pregnant women experience compresses the median nerve in the wrist. There are modifications provided in exercises if this condition affects you. And some exercises (such as the kickback with palm forward) will help carpal tunnel. You can also perform wrist extensions and flexions with a small hand weight. Try not to grip the weight tightly.

BACK PAIN

With your increase in weight and the fact that it is "front loaded," you may begin to experience even greater soreness. If you're unlucky enough (although you're lucky in my book) to have your boobs double and triple in size, you may get more back pain, and pain during exercise. Your core muscles act as a back brace, so back and abdominal strengthening is key, especially if your chest gets rather large. Because you need to do some extra exercises for the traps and lats (your back muscles) if you grow a lot in your chest, here are three exercises you can do a few times a week for a few minutes.

Exercises: Blade, Rotator, Lat pull-down (no weights); 2 sets of 15

- Blade: Activate your core. Touch your fingertips in front of your chest with your elbows parallel. Without arching your back (keep your core activated), pull your arms back as if you are trying to touch your elbows behind you. Squeeze your upper back.
- Rotator: Activate your core. Place your elbows at your hips with forearms pointing to the sides of the room. Without arching your back (keep your core activated), pull your arms back as if you are trying to touch the backs of your palms together behind you. Squeeze the upper/middle back.
- Lat pull-down: Activate your core. Place your arms over your head with your palms forward. Without arching your back, draw your elbows down and slightly behind your hips. Squeeze the middle of your back.

DIASTASIS RECTI

At the latter stages of the second trimester (or at the beginning if you are pregnant with twins), diastasis recti may appear. You will *not* perform the core section of the workout in the second or third trimester if this condition affects you. Refer to page 84 to determine if you have diastasis recti. There are some exercises you can do, which are located in the core section on page 146.

Monday, Wednesday, Friday (Weeks 14–27)

PRE-WORKOUT ACTIVITIES

1. Hydrate and fuel: Drink and eat.
2. Take ten cleansing diaphragmatic breaths: Inhale and exhale through your nose.
3. Clear your mind: Forget your to-do list for now and take some time for yourself.

Reminders during your workout:

1. **Core activation:** See page 92, and the Mandatory Warm-up on page 93.
2. **Perform a Kegel:** Doing Kegels will help maintain a strong pelvic floor. Contract your muscles as if you are cutting off the flow of urine. Hold

this contraction for 10 seconds. Repeat. Remember not to contract the abs, buttocks, or thigh muscles.

3. Take a break when needed.
4. Beginners will do 1 set of 15 of each toning exercise. Veterans will do 2 sets of 15 of each toning exercise with about a 20-second rest between sets.
5. Get your doctor's permission first and *do not* use this book if you are carrying more than two babies.

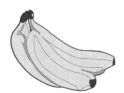

At twenty-one weeks your baby is the size of a banana. Bananas are good for mom as they contain potassium and vitamins C, B_1, B_2, B_6, and E.

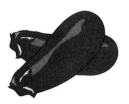

At twenty-five weeks your baby is the size of an eggplant. Eggplant is good for Mom as it is low in calories, high in fiber, and contains vitamins A and C.

Mandatory Warm-up (5 minutes)

Minute 1: Step knee

Target: Raise your heart rate and increase blood flow to your muscles.
Start: Stand with your feet shoulder-width apart.
Motion: Bend your arms at the elbows and make soft fists. Simultaneously lift your right knee and your left arm. Switch and repeat.
Pointers: Quickly raise your legs and arms to increase the effort and raise your heart rate. Stay light on your feet; as you touch down with one foot, immediately raise the other.

Minute 2: Push knees

Target: Raise your heart rate and increase blood flow to your muscles.

Start: Stand with your feet shoulder-width apart.

Motion: Bend your arms at the elbows and make soft fists. Simultaneously lift your right knee and both arms. As you lower your right knee, lower your elbows to your sides and open your hands so that your palms are facing the ceiling. As you raise your left knee, bring both of your arms above your head with your palms still facing the ceiling.

Pointers: Quickly raise your legs and arms to raise your heart rate. Stay light on your feet; as you touch down with one foot, raise the other. Keep your palms up and your shoulders relaxed. Don't scrunch your neck and shoulder muscles. If you're feeling it, let out a *whoo hoo!* on the arm pump.

Minute 3: Quarter squat

Target: Raise your heart rate and increase blood flow to your muscles.

Start: Place your feet shoulder-width (or farther) apart. Put your hands on your hips.

Motion: Inhale as you raise your chin and focus your eyes on a point on the ceiling just ahead of you. Bend your hips and your knees as you lower your butt toward the floor. The lowest you should descend is forty-five degrees. Exhale as you return to the starting position.

Pointers: Keep your hands on your hips throughout the exercise. Keep your knees soft and focus on your breathing. Don't drop your chin or lower your eyes!

Minute 4: Quarter squat and pull

Target: Raise your heart rate and increase blood flow to your muscles.

Start: Place your feet shoulder-width (or farther) apart. Put your hands on your hips.

Motion: Inhale as you raise your chin and focus your eyes on a point on the ceiling just ahead of you. Bend your hips and your knees as you lower your butt toward the floor. Exhale as you return to the starting position. The lowest you should descend is forty-five degrees. Variation: As you squat, pull your elbows toward your hips. Then extend your arms above your head as you stand up.

Pointers: Keep your hands on your hips throughout the exercise. Keep your knees
soft and focus on your breathing. Don't drop your chin or lower your eyes!

Minute 5: Alternating side lunge

Target: Raise your heart rate and increase blood flow to your muscles.
Start: Stand with your toes pointing forward and your feet two to three feet
apart (at least shoulder width).
Motion: Place your hands on your hips. Inhale and, with your knees soft,
shift your weight from your hips to the right. Your left leg should remain
straight and your left foot should stay in full contact with the floor. Exhale
and shift your weight back to center. Pause for a count of two before shifting your weight to the left.
Pointers: As you shift your weight from center, be sure to bend the knee that
will be supporting your weight. You should feel a mild stretch in your inner
thigh and around your hip.

Cardio Block: Optional

See page 137.

Toning Section (12–22 minutes)

If you are a beginner, you will take 12 minutes to finish one set of each exercise. Veterans will take 22 minutes to finish two sets of each exercise. While
these are suggested times, please exercise at your own pace! Veterans, you
have the option of doing two sets with a 20-second rest between or doing 1 set
completing the toning portion, then repeat.

Repetitions: 1 set of 15 for beginners, 2 sets of 15 for veterans.
Note: If you did the optional cardio block, take a minute or two before lowering to the floor for push-ups.

Knee push-ups/"girl" push-ups

Target: Core, deltoids (shoulders), upper back, chest, triceps (back of arms), biceps.
Start: Kneel on the floor. Place your hands on the floor with your face down
and your arms extended. Your hips are also extended. Keep your hands flat
and your head neutral. Align your shoulders above your wrists.

Motion: Keeping your elbows at your sides, bend them to lower your chest to the floor. Keep your body in a straight line from the top of your head to your knees. Do not let your belly touch the floor.

Pointers: Don't arch your back or allow your belly to sway below your hips. Be sure to keep your shoulders directly over your wrists.

Modifications: Instead of doing the exercise on the floor, put your hands on a stair. If you have problems with carpal tunnel syndrome, then use hand weights as a platform to help support your weight: Grip them on the floor as you perform your push-ups.

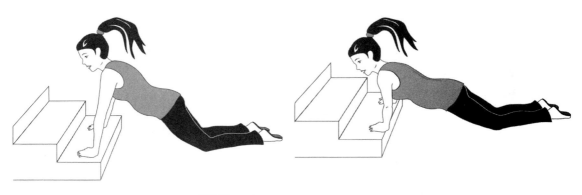

"Girl" push-ups

One-leg squats

Use heavy weights and adjust as you get bigger. Perform 1 set on your right leg, then 1 set on your left leg.

Target: Quadriceps (front of leg), hamstrings (back of leg), glutes (butt), abductors, adductors, core.

Start: Stand with your feet shoulder-width (or slightly farther) apart. Shift your weight onto your right leg and lift your left heel. Hold weights at your sides.

Motion: Flex your hips slightly, then bend your knees to ninety degrees. Most of your weight should be on your right heel. Keep your knees behind your toes. The goal is to sit to ninety degrees and then extend to stand. Keep a neutral spine. Complete one set, then shift your weight onto your left leg and perform another set.

Pointers: Keep your knees behind your toes. Try to bend your knees to a ninety-degree angle.

Modifications: Place your arms at shoulder height in front of you for counter-balance (no weights). If you need more balance, hold on to a sturdy chair. As you get bigger in your second trimester, you'll have your own set of "weights" in your belly for lower-body exercises.

Repetitions: 1 set of 15 for beginners, 2 sets of 15 for veterans.

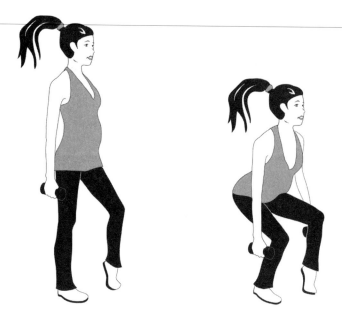

One-leg squats

Posture curls, heavy weights

Target: Biceps, core (abs and back).

Start: Stand with your feet a few inches apart and a weight in each hand. Keep your upper arms and elbows gently pressed against your body for the duration of the exercise.

Motion: With your palms facing out, flex at the elbows and bring the weights up toward your shoulders. Keep a neutral spine.

Pointers: Try not to let your elbows leave your sides, and do not bend at the wrists. Don't swing the weights; slowly raise and lower them.

Modification: If this bothers your carpal tunnel, you can perform the exercise with your palms facing front instead of out to the sides.

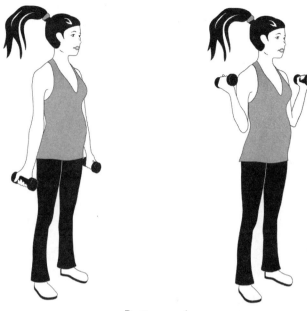

Posture curls

Wide reverse lunge

Use heavy weights and adjust as you get bigger. Perform 1 set on your right leg, then 1 set on your left leg.

Target: Quadriceps (fronts of thighs), hamstrings (backs of thighs), glutes (butt), abductors (outer thighs), adductors (inner thighs), calves.

Start: Stand with your feet twelve to eighteen inches apart. Place weights in your hands with your arms at your sides.

Motion: Step back two to three feet with your right leg. Bend both knees to ninety degrees and slightly flex your hips. Keep a majority of your weight on your front foot and your knee directly over your heel. Then extend both knees and hips to upright position. Perform 1 set on your right leg, then switch.

Pointers: Keep your front knee directly over your ankle. Push through your front heel.

Modifications: Again, you have more "weights" in your belly, so adjust the hand weights accordingly, or place a sturdy chair in front of you and perform the exercise without weights.

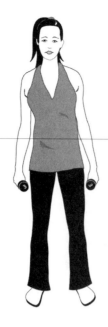
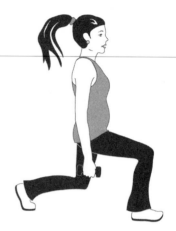

Wide reverse lunge

Do You Have a Lot of Neck Tension?

Try this. While performing the next exercise, watch yourself in the mirror. Do you hunch up or bring your shoulders toward your ears? If so, you will see it in the mirror. Now try to have a long, skinny neck. That will help get rid of some neck tension and make sure you are doing the exercise properly.

Triceps extension, one heavy weight

Target: Triceps (back of arms), deltoids (shoulders), core.

Start: Stand with your feet shoulder-width apart. Hold a weight horizontally with both hands by gripping each end, and extend your arms over your head, keeping them parallel to your ears.

Motion: Keeping your arms next to your ears, bend your elbows so your arms are at a ninety-degree angle. Then extend your arms back up.

Pointers: Keep your upper arms parallel to your ears and think of your elbows as a hinge; they don't move.

Modification: If you are having problems with core activation, sit in a chair as you perform this exercise.

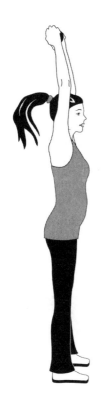 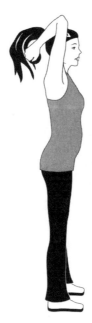

Triceps extension

The Pregnancy Squat

Use the pregnancy squat when picking up a child or other object. Instead of leaning over, keep your core activated by squatting with your legs wide and toes turned out. This will also help your back!

Squat to overhead press, light weights

Target: Quadriceps (front of legs), hamstrings (back of legs), glutes (butt), deltoids (shoulders), triceps (back of arms), core (abs and back).

Start: Stand with your feet shoulder-width (or slightly farther) apart. Extend your arms above your head, holding a weight in each hand, palms facing each other.

Motion: Flex your hips slightly, then bend your knees to a ninety-degree angle. Simultaneously bring the weights down to shoulder height, keeping the ninety-degree angle with your arms. Extend to the standing position and press your arms up, extending your elbows and pushing with your shoulders.

Pointers: Most of your weight should be in your heels, almost lifting your toes. Do not let your knees go past your toes when bending down. Keep your core activated.

Modification: Instead of the overhead press, perform a lateral (side) raise with your arms. Do this by lifting your arms to shoulder height as you squat.

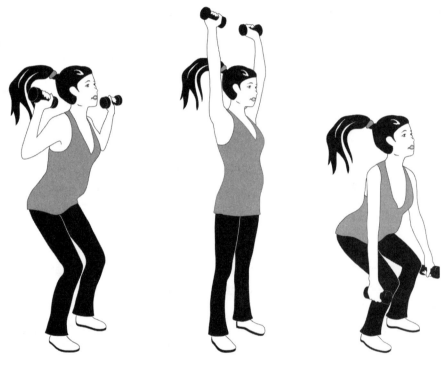

Squat to overhead press

Break and hydrate.

Drink water!

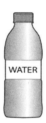

Incline chest press, heavy weights

Use an exercise ball or three pillows to elevate your upper body to a thirty-degree incline.

Target: Chest.

Start: Lie on your back with your head and shoulders elevated. Bring your feet halfway to your butt. Bend your elbows at a ninety-degree angle and bring them up to shoulder height.

Motion: Keep your hands directly above your elbows and squeeze your chest muscles as you extend your arms. Then return to starting position, keeping your elbows at ninety degrees. Maintain a neutral spine.

Pointers: Keep your elbows at a ninety-degree angle. Emphasize the squeeze. Imagine you are squeezing a ball between your breasts.

Modification: Use three pillows under your upper back to prop your upper body on a minimum thirty-degree incline. Do not use an exercise ball in pregnancy if you have never used one before. Your balance is off during pregnancy, and a ball will increase your chances of falling.

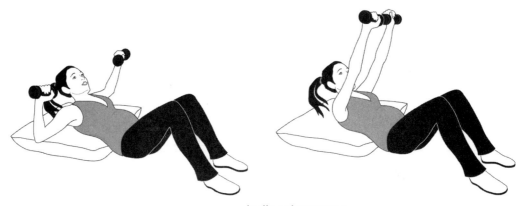

Incline chest press

One-arm reverse fly, light weight

Perform 1 set on your right arm, then 1 set on your left arm.

Target: Upper back (rhomboids, trapezius, lattisimus dorsi), posterior deltoids (back of shoulders).

Start: Stabilize your core with a ninety-degree bend at your hips and your knees flexed. Place your left hand on your left knee. Holding a weight in your right hand, palm facing your body, extend your right arm.

Motion: Raise the weight up and out, away from your body. Do not lock your elbow. Engage your upper-back muscles as your arm rises.

Pointers: Squeeze your shoulder blades together at the top of the lift (you should feel it in the area of where your bra fits). Try not to swing your arm; use your upper back muscles to bring the weight up and then back down.

Modification: Support your upper body as you lean forward by placing the same knee and hand on a sturdy chair to your side.

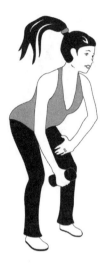 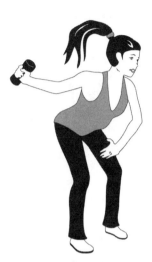

One-arm reverse fly

Curtsy to tap, heavy weights

Perform 1 set on your right leg, then 1 set on your left leg.

Target: Adductors (inner thighs), abductors (outer thighs), glutes (butt), core (abs and back).

Start: Stand with your feet shoulder-width apart. Hold weights in each hand. Shift your weight onto your right leg.

Motion: Extend your left leg one or two feet diagonally behind you and to your right with your heel lifted. Bend your knees to a ninety-degree angle. Return to starting position and tap your left foot.

Pointers: Bend both your knees and keep your front heel on the floor. Do not let your knees go past your toes when bending down. Keep your hips square.

Modification: Use light or no weights, depending on the "weights" in your belly. Advanced modification: Hold one weight with both hands at shoulder height in front of you.

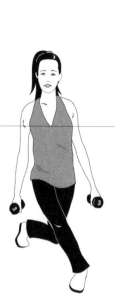
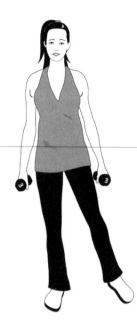

Curtsy to tap

Scapular press with optional plié, light weights

Target: Deltoids (shoulders), upper back (rhomboids, trapezius, latissumus dorsi), core (abs and back).

Start: With a weight in each hand, bend your elbows ninety degrees, raise them to shoulder level, and bring them in front of you with palms facing each other. Optional plié position: Place your feet in a wide stance with your toes turned out forty-five degrees or more.

Motion: Rotate outward at the shoulder joints so that your arms are perpendicular to your body. Your elbows should stay at a ninety-degree angle. Optional: Plié as you squeeze your upper back muscles to swing your elbows out.

Pointers: Keep your abdominals engaged throughout the exercise. Keep your spine aligned.

Modification: Sit in a chair if you find you arch your back easily.

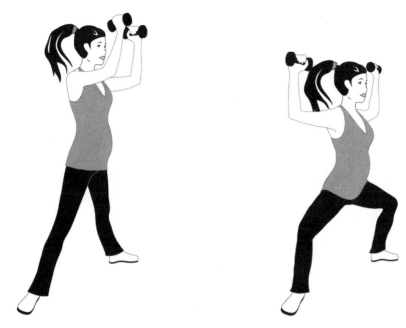

Scapular press with optional plié

Cardio Block

Perform each of the following for 30 to 45 seconds, taking a break in between exercises if necessary.

1. Prego jacks: Jump out to quarter squat and jump in; beginners, do heel digs, which are low-impact jumping jacks without the jumping.
2. Mini-rope: Pretend jump-rope.
3. Lateral ski: Hop sideways from one leg to the other.
4. Push knees: Just like the warm-up but faster.
5. Knees, like in the warm-up.

Yoga Cooldown (8–10 Minutes)

3-minute march in place to cool down. (March slowly; you should be bringing your heart rate down.)

Note: You will hold each pose through five deep yoga breaths. Do not close your eyes since you are pregnant.

Is yoga enough of a workout on its own?

Maybe, but only if you haven't worked out much in the past.

Windshield wiper

- Place your hands on your hips with your feet hip-width apart, knees slightly bent.
- Step back, then hinge at your hips as you sit back, placing a majority of your weight on your back leg.
- Straighten your front leg, flexing your foot toward you.
- With your front foot, perform a motion like a slow windshield wiper. Repeat 4 times.
- Advanced modification: Feel a deeper stretch in your hips by keeping the same position as above, but move your hips side to side like a windshield wiper.

- Beginner modification: Place your hands on a wall in front of you, instead of on your hips.
- Repeat other side.

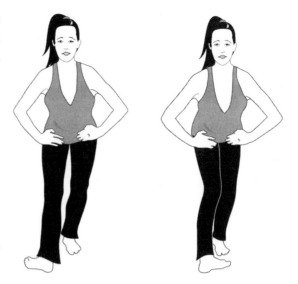

Windshield wiper

Modified single-leg staff

- Take a bath towel and fold it in quarters.
- Grasp both ends of the towel to form a loop.
- Sit with your legs comfortably apart in front of you.
- Bring one foot in toward your midline so that the bottom of your foot is facing your opposite thigh.
- Lean forward from the waist and place the towel around the arch of the foot extended in front of you.
- As you inhale, use the towel to gently pull your head and upper body out over your extended leg.
- Hold for one second and then relax and return to the upright position.
- Repeat for 5 breaths.

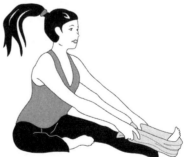

Modified single-leg staff

Butterfly

- Sit with your legs comfortably apart in front of you.
- Bring the soles of your feet together. (Keep them at a distance that is

comfortable for you. You should feel a slight stretch in your groin and upper thighs, but no discomfort.)

- Your knees should be six to twelve inches off the floor.
- Bring your knees down toward the floor in a slow, smooth motion.
- Raise your knees back up to the starting position in a slow, smooth motion.
- Repeat 5 times.

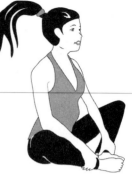

Butterfly

Pigeon open chest (modify with towel under buttocks)

- Start in the butterfly seated position.
- Bend your right knee and swing that leg forward, bringing the knee outside the right hand while straightening your left leg behind you.
- Square your hips toward the floor.
- Use padding under the right side of your butt as necessary to bring your hips square.
- Try the following variations:
  - ◊ Bring your torso down into a forward bend over your right leg.
  - ◊ Let the weight of your body rest on your right leg.
  - ◊ Continue squaring your hips and breathing into the tightness.
  - ◊ Make sure the top of your left foot keeps pressing down into the mat.
  - ◊ Come back up, bringing your hands in line with your hips.
  - ◊ Bend your left knee and reach back for your left foot with your left hand.
  - ◊ Draw your foot toward your butt, stretching your left thigh.
  - ◊ Square your shoulders to the front of the room.
- Repeat pose on the other side.

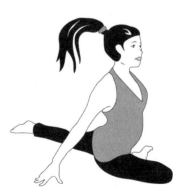

Pigeon open chest

Firm pose

Sit on your heels with your knees bent beneath you. Modify with a towel under your buttocks, then lift your hips from your heels only to the point of comfort as your belly gets bigger.

This is an optional exercise! (All exercises are optional, but with this specific exercise some moms find discomfort.)

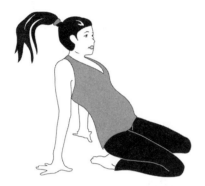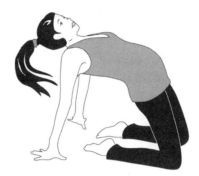

Firm pose

Downward dog

- Come to your hands and knees with your wrists beneath your shoulders and knees below your hips.
- Curl your toes under and push back, raising your hips and straightening your legs.
- Let your head hang, and move your shoulder blades away from your ears and toward your hips.
- Engage your quadriceps strongly to take the weight off your arms, making this a resting pose.
- Rotate your thighs inward, keeping your tail high and sinking your heels into the floor.
- Check that the distance between your hands and feet is correct by coming forward to a plank position. The distance between your hands and feet should be the same in a plank and a downward dog. Do not step your feet toward your hands in downward dog in order to get your heels to the floor. This will happen eventually as your muscles lengthen.

Modification: Use a chair or other raised platform to decrease the amount of distance you have to bend.

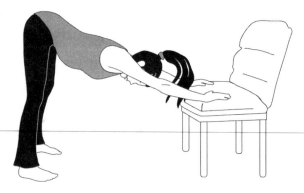

Modified downward dog

Cow to cat pose
Do not do this pose if you have diastasis recti.

- Begin on all fours, with your wrists in line with your shoulders and your knees in line with your hips.
- Keep your spine, neck, and head aligned. Visualize a line extending from your tailbone through the top of your head.
- Inhale and curl your toes under, let your belly drop, and slowly raise your chin toward the ceiling. This is the cow pose.
- Exhale and drop the tops of your feet back to the floor, round your spine, and drop your head and look at your navel. Visualize a cat stretching in a Halloween decoration.
- Repeat the cat to cow stretch on each inhale and exhale for the next five breaths, synchronizing the movement with your breathing.

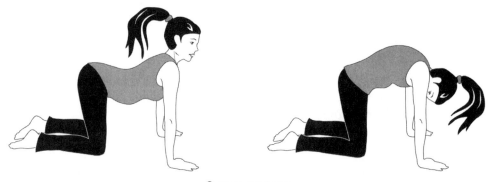

Cow to cat pose

Side angle to supported triangle

- Begin with feet 3½ to 4 feet apart. Point your right toe outward.
- Drop your left heel down to the floor.
- Bend your right knee so your calf and thigh are at a right angle; your thigh should be parallel to the floor.
- Bring your right elbow in toward your right thigh and your left arm up toward the ceiling, opening your chest and stacking your left shoulder on top of your right.
- Straighten your right knee as you exhale and place your right hand on your right leg. Inhale into side angle and repeat 5 times.

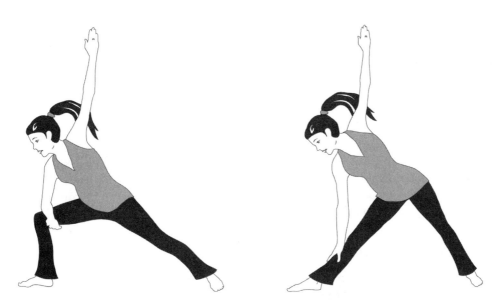

Side angle to supported triangle

Core (4–5 Minutes)

Lindsay's reminder: Please perform the ha-ha-ha until core activation becomes a habit.

Do not do core exercises if symptoms of diastasis recti are present.

Quadruped pelvic tilt

From the cat position in the yoga cooldown, pull your belly button in and tilt the hips so your back rounds slightly. Release to cat position and repeat. **Repetitions:** 1 set of 15.

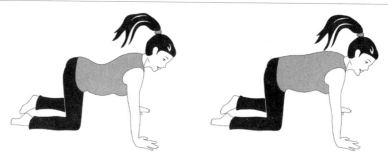

Quadruped pelvic tilt

Plank

Start: Lying on the floor, place your palms on the ground directly under your shoulders. Keep your arms and legs straight as you do a push-up. Pull your navel in so your body forms a straight line from the top of your head to your toes. Try not to let your hips flex. Push the ground away to fully support your upper body.

Pointers: Try to maintain a straight head-to-toe alignment. Imagine wires connected to the top of your head and the soles of your feet pulling you in opposite directions.

Repetitions: Hold this position for 30 seconds.

Teaser swing

Start: Rest on your glutes with your arms extended out to the side.

Motion: Shift your shoulders from side to side, leading with one arm. The farther you lean back and the straighter your arms are, the harder your core has to work to help you maintain balance.

Pointers: Keep your chin tucked to your chest to help you stay steady.

Modification: Lead with your elbow and tap it behind you instead of keeping your arm straight.

Repetitions: 1 set of 12 for beginners; 1 set of 20 for veterans.

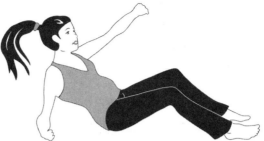

Teaser swing

Single knee-ins in turnout (beginner)
Double knee-ins in turnout (veterans)

Start: Lean back on an incline with your elbows in line with your shoulders and your legs straight.

Motion: Draw your upper back muscles together. Bend your knees to bring your heels close to your body. Let your knees fall open in a turnout. Pull one knee close to your body and raise your toe about six inches off the floor. Bring your knee back down and switch legs. For double knee-ins, keep your knees together and perform the same movement (this will be harder to do as your belly grows).

Repetitions: 1 set of 15.

Veterans, you can also choose to perform the rowboats from the First Trimester Plan (pages 112–113).

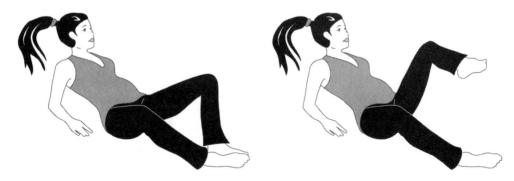

Single knee-ins in turnout

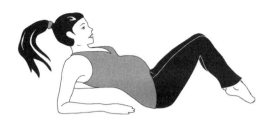 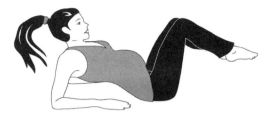

Double knee-ins

DO YOU HAVE DIASTASIS RECTI?

You can perform a few reps of the following exercises:

1. Pelvic clock rotations: Sit on an exercise ball. Your feet should be shoulder- to hip-width apart for balance. While sitting, rotate your hips in a clockwise motion for 5–10 reps, then counterclockwise. The motions should be very small, so that you move only your pelvis. That way you will engage the core, not the legs.
2. Sit on an exercise ball. Walk your feet forward and lean your upper body back slightly. Hold your right side lightly with your left hand as you lean back to the right. Go back only a few inches and release. Switch sides.
3. Squat and pelvic tilt: This is an exercise you will do in your third trimester. You can find it on page 164.

Remember: You should not work on an exercise ball during pregnancy if you've never used one before.

Tuesday (Weeks 14–27)

PREGNANCY CARDIO PENDURANCE WALK (HILLS ARE GOOD)

Intensity	Time	Speed
3–5	5 minutes	warm-up
5–6	1 minute	walk
7–8	1 minute	speed walk
5–6	2 minutes	walk
7–8	2 minutes	speed walk

Intensity	Time	Speed
5–6	3 minutes	walk
7–8	3 minutes	speed walk
5–6	4 minutes	walk
7–8	4 minutes	speed walk
5–6	5 minutes	walk
7–8	5 minutes	speed walk
3–4	5 minutes	cooldown/slow walk

OR

INTERVAL WALK

Intensity	Time	Speed
3–5	5 minutes	warm-up walk
6–8	3 minutes	speed walk
5	2 minutes	walk
6–8	3 minutes	speed walk
5	2 minutes	walk
6–8	3 minutes	speed walk
5	2 minutes	walk
6–8	3 minutes	speed walk
5	2 minutes	walk
6–8	3 minutes	speed walk
5	2 minutes	walk
6–8	3 minutes	speed walk
5	2 minutes	walk
3–4	5 minutes	cooldown/slow walk

Runners

If you have been jogging, you can do it as long as you feel comfortable. Please replace the speed walks with jogging.

Busy Moms and Calorie Burning

Being a busy mom doesn't always translate into burning enough calories to ensure that you are controlling your weight gain. I've said it many times before, but a healthy mom means a healthy family! You make sure your kids have a well-balanced meal and always watch over their health. But of course you forget to watch over your own health. So if you're so busy the drive-through is part of your daily regimen, you are kidding yourself about your health (although it will happen—just don't let it happen daily; refer to page 64 for your "better" fast-food choices). Take the time to take care of you!

Just because you are busy running around does not mean you are burning the appropriate number of calories. Look at running those errands as a bonus burn, not an excuse to consume bad calories. And I may sound a bit like Dr. Phil, but has that strategy of counting your daily activities as a workout worked out for you yet? Chances are it hasn't.

Why is that?

Everyone Can Do It!

I have two great friends who are wonderful examples of the truth that no matter how busy we are, we can find time to work out. My friend Karen runs a StrollerFit camp in St. Louis called Hot Mamas In Training. She is also a wife and full-time mom of two girls, and she works full-time as a registered dietitian at a hospital. How does she manage all this? She told me that at the beginning of every week she pencils in her workouts on her daily planner. Some workouts have to be scheduled in the morning and some after the girls go to bed. Otherwise she won't get them in. The lesson? Plan ahead!

Another friend, Kathryn Sansone, is a mother of ten, an author, and a fitness professional. She has been on a number of TV shows (including *Oprah*), and even with ten kids, she finds time to work out almost every day. She will even jog to lunch with friends in order to fit in a workout! Being flexible and finding ways to fit a workout into your busy schedule requires a bit of ingenuity, but remember, necessity is the mother of invention!

Another group of women I know, from my Stroller Pump class, drop off the older kids at preschool and bring the younger kids to class. By the time they're done with their workout, the kids are ready to be picked up.

· 7 ·

THIRD TRIMESTER EXERCISE PLAN

Weeks 28–38

Pregnant with twins? Weeks fourteen through twenty to twenty-four you will skip the cardio block and all cardio segments. I also ask that you skip the core section. ACOG suggests that women carrying multiples refrain from aerobic exercise, so eliminate the Tuesday workouts, plus the cardio blocks. But, again, do what your doctor says is best, which could be swimming or prenatal yoga *only*.

Wow! Can you believe it? You are about to enter your seventh month of pregnancy. And if you don't feel large and in charge yet, you will very soon! If you're a first-time mom—or even a veteran—and you are feeling like your life is being turned upside down, you aren't alone.

Your baby is also making the transition to life standing—well, OK, floating—on its head. That's a perfectly normal response, since babies are generally born headfirst, and they don't experience any kind of discomfort in that position. They are also aware of light and dark now, and that may have an effect on their activity level and the hours they keep.

Many women report that the third trimester is often the easiest on them mentally—with the exception of the waiting and wondering. You've undergone most of the changes and you've grown accustomed to the majority of them. That may not be the case for all women, but you can at least see the finish line, and that may help to motivate you as you round the final bend. You'll soon be in the delivery room, so here's a preview of what you can expect.

LABOR AND DELIVERY

The first stage of labor can last for several hours: dilation of the cervix, cramping, and labor contractions.

Second stage of labor: pushing and crowning
Third stage of labor: delivery (usually lasts about thirty minutes; more pushing, but less than before)
Fourth stage of labor: rest, repair, relaxation. This final stage is really more about getting back to normal than anything else. Your blood pressure, temperature, and heart rate will stabilize in much the same way a marathon runner's does: a little at a time during the hour after the placenta is delivered.

C-SECTION DELIVERY

The fourth stage was the hardest for me. After my C-section, I started throwing up in the recovery room while *everybody* went to watch Taylor's bath. Otherwise the C-section was not difficult. My only complaint was the swelling from head to toe. And all I wanted to do was get home, away from visitors and nurses waking me up every hour or two. Check out the bikini-cut incision (the doc will not cut through your muscles) on page 176.

Hang in There

At this stage in your pregnancy, you're probably getting more and more uncomfortable. When tying your shoes becomes a workout or carrying your toddler is too much, you know you're approaching the end of your pregnancy. You have insomnia because you're worried about pooping on the delivery table, or you pee every hour during the night, which also messes with your sleep. You tire *very* easily, and all you want is a good night's sleep. I got more sleep after having my first baby than during my third trimester of being pregnant with her (of course, I didn't have a toddler waking me up)!

Sleep and mental health are equally as important as all this fitness stuff. So take care of yourself and your baby. If you didn't get much sleep or you feel exhausted, move right to the yoga portion of this workout. We spend a lot of time on the floor in these exercises to help relieve your legs (which support your extra weight, boobs, and that baby all day long), but it is also important to keep your blood circulating through your legs. Doing this will prevent you from developing some but not all spider veins and reduce swelling. But as I keep saying, exercise is also wonderful for your mental health. Take your ten cleansing breaths and go!

Because of the advanced state of your pregnancy, your workout will decrease in intensity. With the additional weight you are carrying, it is going to take less effort to get to the same working level as in the previous trimesters. Keep in mind all that blood still needs to flow to your baby. So do not push yourself in the third trimester. Many women find it difficult to breathe as easily as before. This is because your baby is growing and pushing your diaphragm up into your chest. Despite that, your breathing capacity is the same and your ribs have expanded to accommodate your growing baby and your growing you. At this stage, you are moving 50 percent more air, which is why exercise is a bit tapered by the third trimester. Use the intensity scale, but also know you may be breathing harder because of your baby getting bigger and taxing your body a bit more. You could be short of breath but not even close to fatigue.

Functional Training

At this stage, in addition to toning we're preparing you for birth and motherhood. You need strength to lug the bundle of joy around, so we're going to do a lot of functional exercises. That means these exercises will help you develop the muscles you need to perform typical daily tasks such as picking up your baby. I've also made allowances for the fact that you have your own "weights" in your belly. I've adjusted the exercises so that you will typically use lighter weights than in the first and second trimesters, but if those lighter weights still seem to be a problem for you, don't use any weights at all.

Combating Back Pain

According to the American Council on Exercise, 50 percent of women will experience lower-back pain. If the only thing supporting your back and your abs is your spine, those sensitive disks and connective tissue are going to be strained during pregnancy. And strain equals pain. But the good news is those women who exercise experience back pain with less frequency and sometimes not at all. I never experienced back pain. All of the workouts you did in the first and second trimesters were choreographed with this in mind, not only to prevent lower-back pain and stay strong for your growing front side, but to strengthen your back for mommyhood.

Also, a strong back leads to a strong core and slimmer waistline. Remember, your back is part of your core and helps bring in the tummy. For that reason, use my strengthening exercises not only to help you now, but to help your body bounce back after giving birth.

Office Exercises

If you work at a desk, it is especially important to do both strengthening and stretching exercises. Try the spinal extension with chair support or spinal flexion from the yoga section (see page 169) to relieve a strained back. Do this at least every hour.

You can also get some exercise by taking the stairs instead of the elevator or getting up for a walk around the office every thirty minutes. Not only will this help prevent swelling, but you can burn a few extra calories if you just don't have the energy to work out.

Pubic pain and round ligament pain are also common in the third trimester, especially if you are expecting your first child. The bones and connective tissues in this area are spreading. It is not harmful, but make sure to ask your doctor if you feel it in excess. Exercise will not make this condition worse. Monitor this and the issues mentioned in Chapter 2, and contact your doctor when you feel you need to.

> Practice taking the arch out of your back and improve your posture with the ha-ha-ha. Engage your transverse: Place one hand on your belly, inhale deeply, and on the exhale say "ha-ha-ha." Notice that as you say those words, the arch disappears. Now you must think about doing this while performing each exercise, which is a challenge at first, but it will become a habit.

How Do I Deal with Urinary Incontinence?

One in three women experiences urinary incontinence when exercising—and that's not one in three pregnant women! Fifty-three percent experience it after their first pregnancy, and 85 percent experience it after subsequent pregnancies.[33] There are two ways to help urinary incontinence before considering surgery: bladder training and pelvic floor exercises. I am going to cover Kegel exercises and "squeeze before you sneeze" to help with urinary incontinence.

PELVIC FLOOR DEVELOPMENT (SQUEEZE BEFORE YOU SNEEZE)

If you are about to cough, sneeze, or strain, it is important to pull your pelvic floor muscles up and in. Brace your muscles before sneezing and you should prevent leakage. Remember, your pelvic floor muscles act as a sling from the pubic bone to tailbone. Pregnancy, childbirth, and decreasing estrogen weaken these muscles—but these muscle fibers can be trained! Like any muscle group, these muscles have to be specifically targeted. You wouldn't swim to train for a marathon, right? So let's find the correct muscles to train.

The Kegel exercises are the best way to identify and isolate your pelvic floor muscles. Remember that in order to strengthen any muscle you have to overload it, meaning you have to work it beyond the point of its previous condition. Doing multiple sets of Kegel exercises while you are driving, watching television, eating, and so on can do wonders to help you maintain control of your bladder.[34]

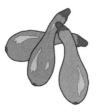

At thirty-one weeks your baby is the size of a squash. Squash is also beneficial to Mom as it is low in calories and contains fiber and vitamins A and C.

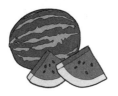

At thirty-seven weeks your baby is the size of a watermelon!

Wow! Watermelon is also beneficial to Mom (especially on a hot summer day), as it is full of water and known to contain antioxidants. It is a powerful fruit full of beta-carotene, vitamins A, C, B_6, and B_1, potassium, and magnesium. And it's also very low in calories!

A Final Note Before You Begin

Remember, exhale on the effort. I will adjust weights for you since you probably have at least thirteen extra pounds on your legs. Your center of gravity has changed, so do the exercises to accommodate for your difference in balance.

Monday, Wednesday, Friday (Weeks 28–38)

Refer to page 123 for pre-workout activities and reminders for your workout.

Mandatory Warm-up (5 minutes)

Refer to page 93 for the mandatory warm-up.

Cardio Block: Optional

See page 165.

Toning Section (12–22 Minutes)

If you did the optional cardio block, take a minute or two before lowering to the floor for push-ups. If you are a beginner you will take 12 minutes to finish one set of each exercise. Veterans will take 22 minutes to finish two sets of each exercise. While these are suggested times, please exercise at your own pace! Veterans, you have the option of doing two sets with a 20-second rest between or doing one set completing the toning section, then repeat.

Repetitions: 1 set of 15 for beginners, 2 sets of 15 for veterans.

Woodpecker push-ups

Target: Core, deltoids (shoulders), upper back, chest (when hands are placed wide), triceps (back of arms), biceps.

Start: Get down on all fours with your back flat and your head neutral. Your hands should be slightly wider than shoulder-width apart.

Motion: Flex your elbows away from your body until your upper arms are at a forty-five-degree angle. Bend at your hips. Do not let your belly touch the floor.

Pointers: A neutral spine and head are very important. Keep your back strong by looking two feet in front of you.

Modifications: Place your hands on a stair. If you have carpal tunnel, use the incline chest press exercise from the second trimester (pages 133–134) in place of this exercise.

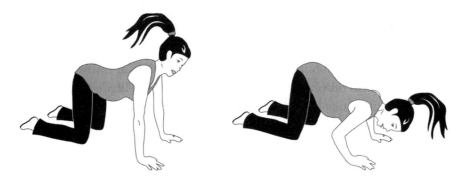

Woodpecker push-ups

Counterbalance squat, one light weight

Target: Quadriceps (fronts of legs), hamstrings (backs of legs), glutes (buncakes), deltoids (shoulders), triceps (backs of arms), core (abs and back).

Start: Stand with your feet shoulder-width (or slightly farther) apart. Extend your arms in front of you at shoulder height, holding a weight with both hands.

Motion: Flex your hips slightly, then bend your knees to a ninety-degree angle. Count to eight slowly. Return to the starting position with your arms still extended in front of you. Count to eight slowly. Repeat.

Pointers: Most of your weight should be on your heels. Your arms stay in counterbalance to help your posture—do not round your shoulders. For core activation, draw your shoulders away from your ears.

Reminder: Do not let your knees go past your toes when bending down. Keep your core activated.

Modification: Place your hands on a sturdy chair in front of you, or place your arms in front of you without weights as shown below.

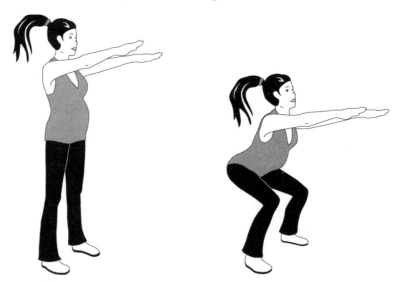

Counterbalance squat

Palm tree, light weights

Target: Core, deltoids (shoulders).

Start: Stand with your feet wider than shoulder-width apart. Slightly flex your hips and knees and bend at the waist. Extend one arm overhead, palm down, while extending your other arm close to your body with your palm up.

Motion: Switch arm positions while keeping a neutral spine.

Pointers: Keep your head and spine neutral. Keep your core activated. Make sure to bring your top arm all the way past your ear. Don't hunch your shoulders.

Modification: Sit in a chair to perform these exercises.

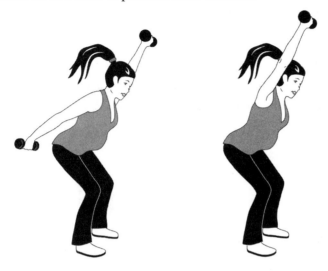

Palm tree, light weights

Balance

To help your balance, widen your stance when performing lunges and squats. Or you can hold on to a sturdy chair or wall.

Lunge and press

Use one heavy weight. Perform 1 set on your right leg, then 1 set on your left leg.

Target: Quadriceps (front of thighs), hamstrings (back of thighs), glutes (butt), abductors (outer thighs), adductors (inner thighs), calves, deltoids (shoulders), core.

Start: Place one weight in your right hand close to your body. Stand with your feet a foot to a foot and a half apart.

Motion: Step back two to three feet with your right leg. Bend both your knees to ninety degrees and slightly flex your hips. Keep a majority of your weight on your left foot while keeping your knee directly over your heel. Reach your right hand toward your left foot as you bend your knees into the lunge. Then extend both knees and hips to the upright position, simultaneously flexing your right elbow and extending your hand overhead. Perform 1 set on your right leg, then switch.

Pointers: Be sure to keep your head above your heart. Perform the exercise slowly.

Modifications: Place a sturdy chair on your left side when working your right leg, and perform the exercise without the weight.

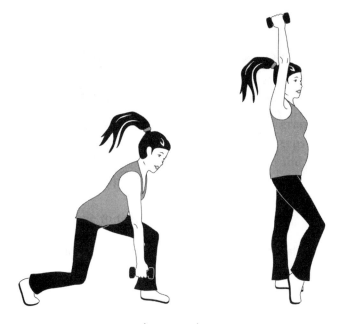

Lunge and press

One-arm triceps extension, one light weight

Target: Triceps (back of arms), deltoids (shoulders), core.

Start: Stand with your feet shoulder-width apart. Holding a weight in your right hand, extend your right arm over your head, so it is parallel to your ear.

Motion: Keeping your arm next to your ear, flex your elbow so that your arm creates a ninety-degree angle. Then extend your arm back up.

Pointers: Keep your upper arms parallel to your ears and think of your elbows as a hinge: They don't move.

Modification: If you are having problems with core activation, sit in a chair as you perform this exercise.

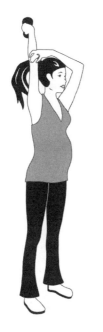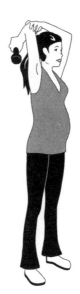

One-arm triceps extension

V-plié (optional), light weights

Target: Deltoids (shoulders), upper back (rhomboids, trapezius, latissumus dorsi), core.

Start: Place your feet wide, with your toes turned out forty-five degrees or more. Hold a weight in each hand with your palms facing your body and your arms hanging straight in front of you.

Motion: Use your upper back to bring your palms in line with your shoulders. Your arms stay straight. Simultaneously bend both knees into a plié squat.

Pointers: Don't swing the weights. Lift and lower them with control. Keep your arms straight.

Modification: Don't do the plié; just work the arms.

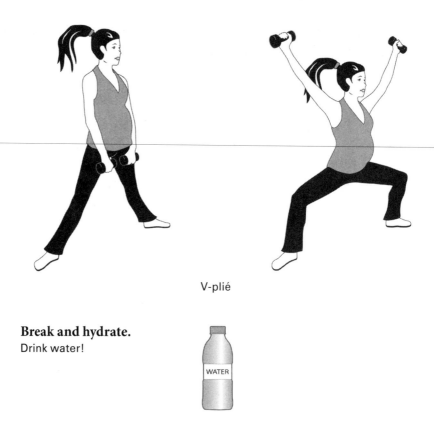

V-plié

Break and hydrate.
Drink water!

Alternating reverse wide lunge, light weights optional

Target: Quadriceps (front of thighs), hamstrings (back of thighs), glutes (butt), abductors (outer thighs), adductors (inner thighs), calves.

Start: Place weights in your hands with your arms close to your body. Stand with your feet twelve to eighteen inches apart.

Motion: Step back two to three feet with one leg. Bend both your knees to ninety degrees and slightly flex your hips. Keep a majority of your weight on your front foot while keeping your knee directly over your heel. Then extend both knees and hips to upright position. Switch legs.

Pointers: Keep your front knee directly over your ankle. Push through your front heel.

Modifications: Again, you have more "weights" in your belly, so adjust the hand weights accordingly, or place a sturdy chair in front of you and perform the exercise without weights.

Refer to the illustrations for the wide reverse lunge (page 129). You will be alternating your legs for 1 complete set of 20.

Hammer to press, heavy weights

Target: Biceps, deltoids (shoulders), triceps (back of arms), upper back, core.

Start: Stand with your feet shoulder-width apart. Extend your arms close to your body. Palms face each other.

Motion: Keeping your palms facing each other, bring the weights to your shoulders, then extend your arms overhead. Bring the weights back to your shoulders, then return to starting position.

Pointers: Keep your knees soft so your body does not swing. Perform the exercise slowly and exhale when you raise your arms overhead.

Modification: Change the overhead press to a side raise. Perform the hammer curl (bend your elbows), then release and extend your arms to your sides to perform a side raise.

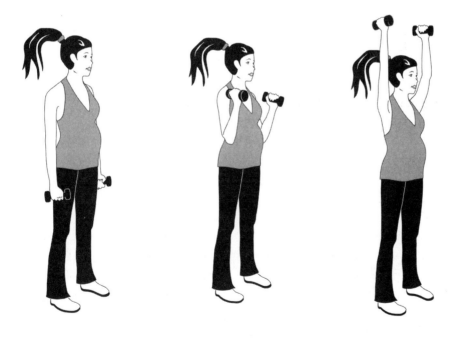

Hammer to press

Stationary side lunge, light weights optional

Target: Quadriceps (front of legs), hamstrings (back of legs), glutes (booty), core, deltoids (shoulders), triceps (back of arms), abductors (outer thighs), adductors (inner thighs), calves.

Start: Stand with your feet shoulder-width apart and the weights close to the body.

Motion: Step to the side with your right leg, keeping your toes pointing straight ahead. Bend your right leg to ninety degrees. Keep your knee behind your toes. Your left leg should stay straight. Then straighten your right leg, keeping your feet in place. Perform one set on your right leg, then one set on your left leg.

Pointers: Protect your knee by keeping it behind your toe as you bend your leg.

Modification: Place your hands on your hips and don't use weights.

To increase the difficulty of this exercise, perform a moving side lunge: Step the right leg in after each lunge. You can also hold heavy weights.

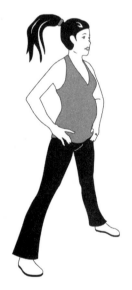 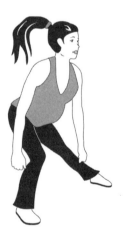

Stationary side lunge

Row to kickback, one light weight

Target: Core, triceps (back of arms), deltoids (shoulders).

Start: Place your feet shoulder-width apart and flex your hips and knees slightly. Keep a neutral spine and place your left hand on your left knee for support. Hold one weight in your right hand and extend your arm with your palm facing forward.

Motion: Flex your right elbow to ninety degrees close to your hip. Then extend your right arm. Flex once again and then return to starting position. Perform one set on your right arm, then one set on your left arm.

Pointers: Lift your elbow higher to make exercise more difficult. Keep your core activated.

Modification: Place your left knee and left hand on a sturdy chair to perform the exercise. This helps with balance and core activation.

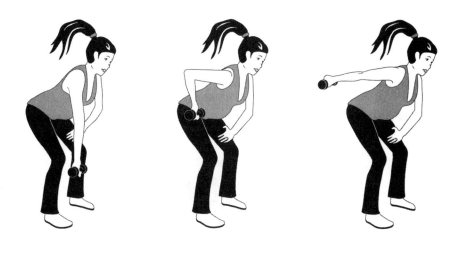

Row to kickback

Squat and pelvic tilt, or "lift and hug the baby"

For this exercise you can use light weights, depending upon your strength level. Use one weight in each hand.

Target: Quadriceps (front of legs), hamstrings (back of legs), glutes (butt), abductors (outer thighs), adductors (inner thighs), pelvic floor, core.

Start: Stand with your back against a wall and your feet one to two feet away from the wall.

Motion: Use your pelvic floor to pull your hip bone toward your baby. Your spine will flatten against the wall. Simultaneously flex your knees forty-five to ninety degrees. Hold that position for a few seconds and stand up.

Pointers: Place a rolled-up towel behind your lower back to make the movement easier.

Modification: Squat only to forty-five degrees or less.

Advanced modification: To make the exercise more difficult, straighten one arm overhead with one light weight so it touches the wall behind you, then switch arms. Release the squat.

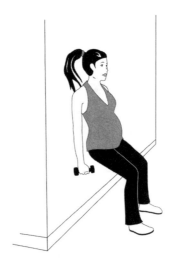

Squat and pelvic tilt

Cardio Block

Perform each of the following for 30 seconds, taking a break in between exercises if necessary.

1. Prego jacks: Jump out to quarter squat and jump in.
2. Mini-rope: Pretend jump-rope.
3. Lateral ski: Hop sideways from one leg to other.
4. Push knees: Just like the warm-up but faster.
5. Stairs or knees, like in the warm-up.

EXPRESS WORKOUT

For the days you just can't commit at least fifteen minutes, I've created a fifteen-minute routine for you.

Warm-up: 1 minute step knee, 1 minute knee pushes, 1 minute quarter squat and pull

Toning: Counterbalance squat, palm tree, V-plié, hammer to press, squat and pelvic tilt (beginners perform 15 of each exercise; veterans perform 15 of each exercise and repeat)

Cardio block: Same as page 104

Cooldown: Walk around your house for a few minutes

Core: Plank (1 set of 20 seconds)

Yoga Cooldown (8–10 Minutes)

Three-minute march in place to cool down (march slowly; you should be bringing your heart rate down)

Note: You will hold each pose through five deep yoga breaths. Do not close your eyes since you are pregnant.

Windshield wiper

Perform this exercise just as you did in the first and second trimesters (pages 107–108), but put your hands against the wall for balance.

Triceps and IT band stretch

- Stand with your feet shoulder-width apart and your hands at your sides.
- Cross your right foot in front of the the left.
- Raise your right arm above your head close to and parallel to your ear.
- Drop your hand behind your back, keeping your elbow lifted.
- Grasp your elbow with your left hand.
- Gently tug your elbow across your body and slightly down.
- As you stretch the back of your arm, tilt your body to the left side, feeling the stretch along the outside of your leg.
- Switch legs and arms and repeat.

Modified pigeon

- Place a towel on the floor under where your buttocks would be. Lower yourself while you bring your arms to the floor, supporting your upper body.
- Let your back knee rest on the floor. Curl your front leg so that your heel is facing the center of your body, and sit on the towel. Lean your torso forward and rest your hands on the floor to the inside of your lead leg.

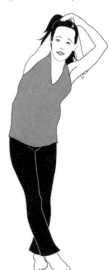

Triceps and IT band stretch

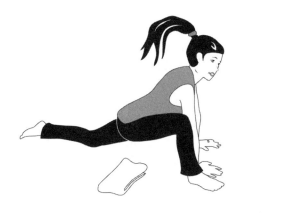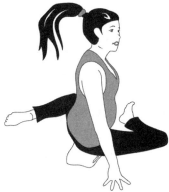

Lunge to modified pigeon

Knee rock

- Sit on your rolled towel or pillow with your legs in front of you, slightly bent.
- Bring one leg toward your midline, using your hands to gently pull your heel closer to your crotch.
- Support your bent leg with one hand underneath your shin and the other around your heel.
- Gently raise your leg, feeling the stretch through your hip, inner thigh, and back of the leg.
- Switch legs and repeat.

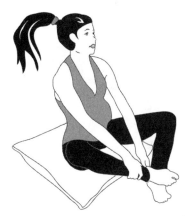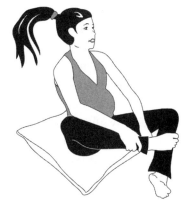

Knee rock

One-leg staff with twist

- Begin in the seated position on your cushion.
- Position your legs in front of you and spread them in a wide V.
- Place your right foot flat on the floor; bring that heel toward your body so that your knee is perpendicular to the floor.
- Place your right elbow inside the raised knee.
- Gently push your knee to the outside while turning your head to the left side.

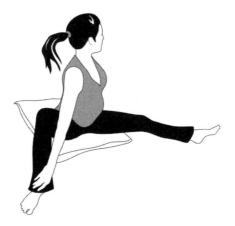

One-leg staff with twist

Seated birth pose

- Sit on the floor (if possible) or on your pillow.
- Extend your legs so that they are in a wide V (just outside your hips).
- Simultaneously bring your knees up toward you.
- Place your hands on your knees.
- Gently tug your knees toward your chest, with your feet coming slightly off the floor.
- Keep your spine aligned and maintain your balance.

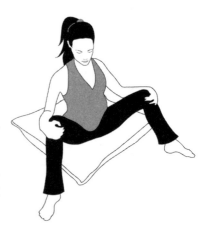

Seated birth pose

Spinal extension with chair support *or* spinal flexion from chair

Do whichever feels better on your body.

Spinal extension with chair support

- Kneel in front of an armchair with your knees spread in a wide V.
- Raise your hands over your head as you tilt forward from your waist.
- Rest your hands on the arms of the chair.
- Keep your head and spine aligned.

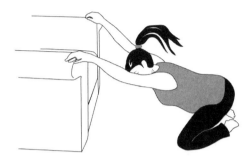

Spinal extension with chair support

Spinal flexion from chair

- Sit on a chair or couch with your legs spread in a wide V and your arms at your sides.
- Point your toes to the outside.
- Gently lower your arms and shoulders between your legs.
- Rest your hands on the floor just inside your feet.
- Slowly raise yourself to the starting position.

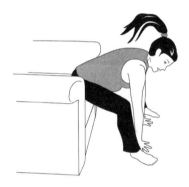

Spinal flexion from chair

Core (3–5 minutes)

Lindsay's reminder: Please continue to perform the ha-ha-ha to activate your core! **Do not do core exercises if you have diastasis recti.**

Half Pilates roll-down

Start: Sit on your glutes with your arms and legs extended in front of you.
Motion: Bend your knees and let them fall open while keeping your feet on the floor. Slowly curve your spine and lean back, looking at your belly button.

Pointers: Only go as far back as you feel comfortable before coming back into sitting position.

Modification: Use an exercise band. Place a handle in each hand and the middle of the band under your feet for added support.

Repetitions: Beginners perform 1 set of 10; veterans perform 1 set of 12.

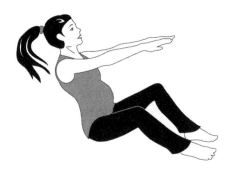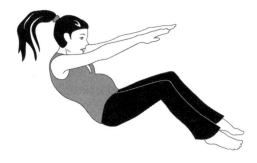

Half Pilates roll-down

Veterans, if you have an exercise ball at home you can perform 20–25 crunches on the ball.

Knee switch

Start: Sit on your glutes. Lean back and rest your elbows on the floor with your palms on the ground to either side of you and your hips slightly bent.

Motion: Bend your knees and flex your hips. Keeping your knees together, rock them from one side to the other while keeping your toes on the floor.

Advanced modification: Keep your toes slightly off the floor.

Repetitions: 1 set of 15.

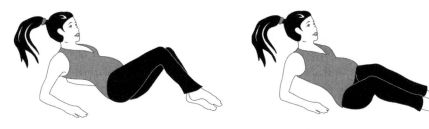

Knee switch

Quadruped arm and leg reach

Start: Place your hands and knees on the
   floor and pull your navel in.
Motion: Extend one leg straight behind
   you and your opposite arm straight in
   front of you.
Repetitions: Hold this position for 10
   seconds. Alternate arm and leg, holding each pose for 10 seconds.

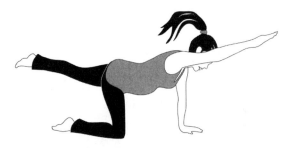

Quadruped arm and leg reach

Tuesday (Weeks 28–38)

PREGNANCY CARDIO INTERVAL WALK

Intensity	Time	Speed
3–5	5 minutes	warm-up walk
6–8	2 minutes	speed walk
5	2 minutes	walk

Repeat two-minute speed walk/two-minute walk 5–6 times followed by a five-minute cooldown/slow walk.

*Remember, in your third trimester you will climb to a 6–8 in intensity much faster due to the hard work your body is doing as the baby gets bigger.

The Final Weeks' Workout

WEEKS 38–40

- 20-minute walk, no intervals

- Yoga poses (see below)
  - ◊ Move through these slowly and concentrate on your breath. I want you to inhale for a count of six and exhale for an eight count. Repeat each 4 times.
  - ◊ This series of yoga poses will bring blood flow to the uterus.

Seated birth pose (on pillow)

Follow the instructions on page 168, but use your cushion.

Inclined goddess pose

Incline at least thirty degrees, (eighteen to twenty-four inches), using a large pillow or two to three small pillows.

- Lie on your back with your head resting on the pillows and your legs extended in front of you.
- Bring your heels toward your midline and bend your knees like a frog's.

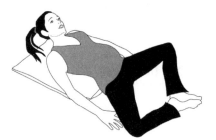

Inclined goddess pose

Yin and yang (on pillow)

- Begin in the seated position with your legs extended in front of you.
- Bring your heels toward your midline and loosely cross them.
- While bringing your heels in, place one arm on top of your belly and the other cradling below it.
- Switch arms.

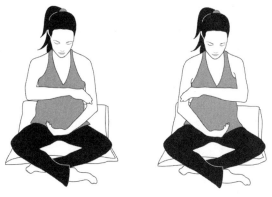

Yin and yang

Around the clock

- Stand with your feet spread beyond shoulder width and your knees bent close to 90 degrees.
- Raise your arms to your sides.
- Bend to one side and rest your arm on your thigh.
- Bring the opposite arm up and over your head.
- Return to the center position and rest both forearms on your thighs.
- Drop your head and look at the floor directly beneath you.
- Bend to your other side, repeating the arm movement.

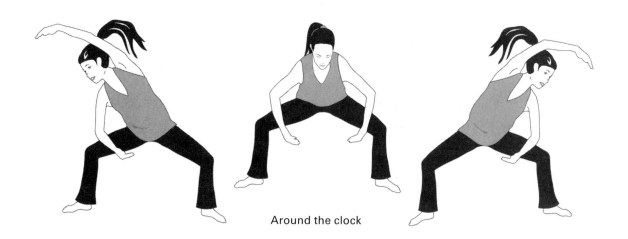

Around the clock

How to Choose a Jogging Stroller

So why is this in the pregnancy section? You might be deciding on which stroller to buy, or if buying two strollers is in your future, this should help you decide. Buying a stroller can sometimes feel like buying a new car, and in some ways that's good. Not only is the decision an important one, but the focus you put on it will take your mind off other worries and concerns.

Many strollers on the market today double as a jogging stroller and a travel system (the infant car seat can move from stroller to car).

Seat and safety

- Look for a five-point harness to keep your child secure.
- Kids love lap trays, and moms love them too—the tray keeps the child from wanting to get out of the stroller.
- Look for a reclining seat for a younger baby.

Easy folding

- Is it light enough to lift into your trunk?
- Can you fold the stroller by yourself?

Tires vs. plastic wheels

- Jogging strollers are made with tires. Some have a fixed front tire, while others have a tire that swivels but can be locked in a fixed front position.
- Wheel sizes are different. Smaller wheels are for smooth surfaces and don't let you move as fast. A majority of strollers have plastic wheels and do no move as easily.
- Tires are much easier to push than platsic wheels, and they make for a smoother ride.

Storage

- We all love our storage, especially cup holders! A lot of European strollers just don't offer as much storage space. Some strollers are made with cup holders and/or extra storage. Are the cup holders deep enough for bottled water?

- These extras are sometimes offered as bags you can Velcro to the stroller.

Do I need a jogging stroller?

- You can easily walk and jog outside without a jogging stroller. But a jogging stroller makes for a smoother and easier push for Mom.
- Some higher-end strollers can be used as both, but the wheels are a bit smaller compared to a jogging stroller.

The Big Day

On the big day, the exercises you have been doing will come in handy! The TA, which has been supporting your baby's weight throughout your pregnancy, will now act like a tube of toothpaste squeezing the baby out. And all the hard work of labor will be followed by some even more challenging work: caring for a newborn and getting your body back.

Pack your bags early, because that big day can arrive at any time! Your doctor should have a list of items to prepare you for your hospital stay. If you are delivering vaginally you will stay two to three days. If you are having a C-section, you will spend between four and five days in the hospital. Of course, if you are delivering in your own home with a midwife, your midwife will prepare you.

One small piece of advice I have for you: Walk around the hospital once you are allowed to get up and move—but only once your doctor gives the OK. This will help prevent postpartum swelling. They've pumped you full of fluids, especially if you were in labor for hours. The same thing goes here as it did in your pregnancy—you must move to reduce swelling. Peeing is another way to reduce swelling, so be sure to drink your water!

I am sure you have prepared yourself in a number of ways for the big day. And if you plan on having your baby vaginally, here are a few labor poses to help with your delivery.

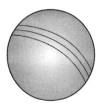 Use assistance when using the ball

- Kneel on all fours and place your chest on the exercise ball. Let your arms hang or hug the ball. This will help alleviate pain in your wrists. Your partner can massage your lower back when you are in this position.
- Standing, place the ball against the wall and lean forward on the ball. This will increase pelvic rotation. Your partner can also give you a back massage when you are in this position.
- Standing, place the ball against the wall and lean your back against the ball. This will provide pressure for your aching lower back.
- Sit on the ball with your legs wide. Sway your hips for relief.

Interested in Lamaze? Lamaze is a registered trademark of Lamaze International, Inc. For more information visit lamaze.org or call 800-368-4404.

THE C-SECTION

IS A BIKINI-CUT C-SECTION REALLY UNNOTICEABLE? AND DOES THE DOC CUT MY MUSCLES?

A Cesarean section is a surgical procedure, so there will always be some scarring, but unlike what most women think, with the exception of the uterus, your doctor will not be cutting through muscle. When a C-section is performed, two sets of abdominal muscles are separated from one another, but they are *not* cut. A transverse (horizontal) cut—the so-called bikini cut—actually causes fewer complications. Since it is below your bikini line, it will be far less noticeable than a longitudinal (vertical) incision.

Many, many moms have approached me asking how my "natural birth" went. I guess because of what I do some women assume I went for the natural option. Well, I decided long ago that drugs were the way for me to go! But both kids were born via C-section; Taylor was lying sideways and Rylan was an emergency.

I met a very strong mom through my fitness videos, and she did opt for natural birth. Her name is Tiffany; she is the mother of four and eagerly gets her body back between pregnancies. She is healthier than ever and feels great! Here is her story about natural delivery, *without* medications:

BIRTH STORY OF MACEY JOY

Weight: 6 lbs 3 oz
Length: 20 inches

Macey was my third pregnancy. My first two children were born without the use of medications. It was very painful and uncomfortable, and labor and delivery was what I dreaded the most with this third baby. I didn't want to go through the excruciating agony of childbirth again. But I also did not want to have medications. I was really interested in finding a way to lessen my pain level so I would be better able to tolerate it. I started researching HypnoBirthing (the Mongan Method). I had heard of HypnoBirthing before, but really didn't know what it entailed. I knew people had "pain-free" or more relaxed childbirth when using this method.

I was very interested in using HypnoBirthing. I found a girl who taught classes in my area, and I was so excited to learn more. I completed the course and practiced using the techniques I learned on a regular basis before my baby was due to be born.

On the night of October 8, I started having some small contractions. They weren't very intense, but they were strong enough to keep me from sleeping that night. I continued to have them the following day, accompanied by some bloody show (blood-tinged mucus—a sign of true labor) with no more intensity than the night before. That evening, around ten p.m., I started to feel more intense contractions. I began using the HypnoBirthing techniques. By two thirty a.m., I decided it was time to go to the hospital. I continued to use the breathing techniques to relax and not fight the contractions, but rather let my body do as it was designed to do. My husband and I made it to triage at the hospital, and by four o'clock I was five centimeters dilated. I had informed the nurses that I was having a HypnoBirthing birth and that I preferred to have the lights low, and to "do my own thing." I wanted it as quiet as possible and wanted to be left with my husband. The nurses were very respectful and encouraged me to do what I needed to do. They left my husband and me alone in the room and let me know they would monitor me from the nurse's station. They also explained how to unhook myself from the monitors if I needed to use the bathroom.

I continued to use my breathing techniques to induce relaxation and progress my labor. My husband also helped by giving me light-touch massage and encouraging me to relax through the contractions. The funny part about this was that with my two previous labors, I couldn't stand to be touched. The pain was so severe that having him even touch my leg to help did the opposite. It made the pain more intense and frustrated me. It was so different this time. I was completely relaxed through the contractions and in between. I was still able to feel the pain, but with much less intensity. I was so much more able to "control" myself throughout labor.

The baby's heart rate was dropping with each contraction and had been doing so since I had arrived at the hospital. Around five thirty a.m., one of the nurses came into the room and said the baby's heart rate was starting to concern them. She asked if I was feeling any pressure; I told her I was feeling a little bit with each contraction. She asked if she could check my progression. I agreed and she reported that I was nine centimeters dilated. My husband and I looked at each other in shock! I said to the nurses, "This is a completely different experience than my first two." With my other children, by the time I was dilated nine centimeters, I was shaking uncontrollably, saying how I couldn't do it anymore, and I was in so much pain! This time, I was in complete control, with a smile on my face. I continued to breathe successfully through each intense contraction.

My water finally broke during one of my contractions. As soon as I finished breathing through the contraction, I told my husband to grab the nurses because my water had broken and I needed to push. The nurses came running in. We had discussed earlier that I would not be waiting for my doctor to deliver the baby, so they quickly checked me and told me to push whenever I wanted to. I birthed my baby on my side at first and then up in a partial squat position to help her to come down the birth canal. They asked my husband if he wanted to help deliver the baby (since my doctor was still ten minutes away) and he eagerly put on gloves.

I pushed for ten minutes and Macey Joy was born, delivered by a nurse and her father. They clamped the cord and my husband cut it. It was only after Macey was placed on my stomach and had been there for several minutes that my doctor walked into the room.

I was so grateful for the nurses who helped me during my labor and delivery. They were wonderful and supportive, letting me have the birth I wanted. They let me do what I wanted and were wonderful. This was by far my best birth! I was amazed at how well the breathing and relaxation techniques worked to help me allow my body to go through the process of birth that it is meant to. It was an incredible experience and I hope to use the same techniques if I have another child.

Becoming a Mother Through Adoption

I became friends with Lisa when we were both St. Louis Rams Cheerleaders. And at the time I had no idea we would have so much in common that didn't have to do with fitness or dancing. I admire Lisa not only because she finds time to own and run a dance studio, is captain of the St. Louis Rams Cheerleaders, and is a very caring individual, but because of her courage to become a mother. Lisa and Greg, like David and me, endured the long, emotional process of in-vitro fertilization. And after many failed cycles and a miscarriage they looked forward to adopting. This is her rewarding story of becoming a mom to Taylor (who was the cutest lil' Rams Cheerleader!).

A few years ago, Lisa and her husband made the biggest decision of their lives: to adopt a child. In the beginning, there were so many questions, and the first step seemed so frightening. After finding an agency to work with, they filled out the endless amounts of paperwork and became "active." Soon, Lisa and Greg were notified of a possible situation. With much excitement, they prepared the nursery for their newborn and anxiously waited. A few days before they were to meet their new baby, they received a phone call stating that the birth mother had changed her mind and had decided to keep her baby. Lisa and Greg felt that their dreams had been crushed. They knew in their hearts that adoption was the answer and that they had to stay strong; it wasn't going to be an easy road.

Several months later, Lisa and Greg were matched with another birth mother, only to have the same thing happen. Although it was difficult to remain hopeful, Greg reminded Lisa that there was a special baby out there just for them and encouraged her to be strong. After only a few weeks, they received their third phone call. They spoke with the birth mother with the hope of talking again soon. Later that day, the agency called and said that the birth mother was in labor, so Lisa and Greg packed their bags and drove for hours.

During the drive, the agency called and said that their baby girl had been born and the birth mother couldn't wait to meet them. They drove straight to the hospital and met the birth mother, a beautiful young girl, who then introduced them to their new daughter. Lisa and her husband knew that this was the baby they were meant to have. It was bittersweet—someone else was hurting by giving up the baby she loved, while Lisa and Greg were getting the baby they had longed for.

The next few days were very challenging as they waited for the birth mother's rights to be terminated. The couple let their faith in God and each other help them through. After a few days, the baby was theirs. They had finally found each other!

"When I look into her bright and beautiful blue eyes, kiss her chubby little cheeks, and feel her warm hugs as she says, 'Mama,' I know that adoption was the best decision we ever made. So my advice to anyone looking to adopt is to stay strong and know in your heart that there is a baby out there waiting for you to find them."

Adoptive mothers and birth mothers face similar challenges when it comes to finding time to work out and eat right. No matter how a child comes into your life, you will face challenges that you need to overcome, but as Lisa's and Tiffany's stories demonstrate, the challenge is always worth the effort!

PART II

Post-Pregnancy

· 8 ·

GETTING YOUR BODY BACK

A Quick Rundown on Nutrition

You've entered what is probably the most challenging phase of your life. Whether you've just given birth to your first and are trying to get used to having a baby who is dependent on you, or you just had your eighth child and have a lot to handle, it's a truly amazing miracle that just happened. As you cringe at the cellulite on the backs of your thighs (which you couldn't spin around to see in the mirror with a big ol' belly), just realize it's only temporary! As you know, I don't want you to think of exercise for the first four weeks. You will train your pelvic floor every other day with three movements. That's it.

I am going to ask you to do some pelvic floor movements the first six weeks of your recovery, starting a few days out. Don't worry, it will take just a few minutes. And it's not considered exercise so much as it is re-engaging your muscles. By doing these movements, along with the pregnancy workouts you already did, you will have your body back within five months—and maybe an even better body! So don't put this book down to collect dust over the next eight weeks—glance forward and think about using your muscles again.

I will make this plain and simple. **If you don't use your core muscles, how do you expect them to return to their pre-pregnancy size?** So exercise is simply a "have to." You *must* spend time on your body—you gave it to another being for the past nine months.

The other component of fitness is, of course, nutrition. What you put into your body post-pregnancy is as important as what you do to get it back into shape. Obviously your priority in the first four weeks is taking care of your baby and making the necessary adjustments to your lifestyle now that you have a new life in your house. That doesn't mean that the good things you were doing in terms of consumption and choices should go out the window—don't throw out your goals and discipline with the baby's bathwater! Sure, you need to treat yourself well, but that doesn't have to mean indulging in food. If you let these first four weeks go by with limited exercise (which you should) and a complete relaxation of your nutritional discipline, you're going to have to work that much harder down the line.

I know you're thinking you cannot possibly fit one more thought into your brain, so I'm going to make it super easy. No grocery lists; no strict meal plans. Eat how you normally eat, with a few rules.

Because I know how busy you are and how many other things are on your mind, I don't want to overload you with all kinds of nutrition information. This chapter is intended to be one you can dip into and out of quickly—kind of like grazing in the kitchen, but I don't want you to do that; do it here instead! With a mix of tips, meal plans, and other information that you need, I'm sure you'll find something that will help make your transition easier.

How Do the Stars Do It?

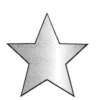

The frenzy of attention over celebrities having babies has died down. I guess we've all realized that they are human too! But what hasn't died down, and probably never will, is all the fuss over how quickly they seem to regain their form once they have had children. Well, if you have the resources and can devote as much time and energy to the project as they are able to (and often have to because how they look is intimately connected with doing their job), here's a quick rundown of the steps you can take to get it done Hollywood-style:

Hire a chef to prepare all your healthy, low-fat meals. Hire a personal trainer to come to your house to whip you into shape during and after your pregnancy. Have an elective C-section and tummy tuck a couple of weeks before your due date to keep from gaining those extra pounds. Hire a great hairstylist, a personal stylist, a and makeup artist to get you looking amazing for your first photos with baby.

You've probably heard of the cleanses, C-section/tummy tucks, elimination of white foods, eating baby food, macrobiotic, two-a-days, breast-feeding filters and machines . . . and the list goes on. And if a celeb got her body back in less than three months, she may have dabbled in one of these or trained five or six days a week for two to three hours a day with a very restricted diet.

Sure, a nutritional cleanse will do the trick, but that is only temporary. Then it wreaks havoc as you pile on extra fat pounds, and fast!

Eliminating all white foods and carbs—that'll do the trick, but how fun is that? And how long can you sustain not eating any sugar, bread, pasta, and potatoes? And can we talk about the permanent bad mood you would be in?

Macrobiotic? Well, if that's your thing.

And breast-feeding . . . yes, you can eat more while you're breast-feeding (I personally enjoyed that), but there is no reason to filter the breast milk or have a breast pump attached to you all day long just so you can savor a few more calories.

Rapid weight loss after having a baby is simply not a good idea. Any doctor will tell you that!

I don't want to leave you with the impression that movie stars and models don't work hard to maintain their great bodies or to regain them after pregnancy. It's just the opposite: Celebrities work very hard at it, because it's part of their job, and they have the time and resources available to clear their schedules so they can go after their workouts as worry-free as possible. They do have to physically do the work, although we all wish there was an invention that burned the calories for us!

For a more realistic approach, see the following steps.

Step 1

You put on anywhere from fifteen to fifty pounds (and hopefully not much more than that!) over the past nine months. Give yourself a break—that is a lot of weight to put on within nine months.

Step 2

Once you are given the OK by your doctor, begin exercising. Start with Phase 1 (page 212).

Step 3

Turn off the pregnancy eating radar—unless you are breast-feeding. Breast-feeding your baby will help you burn extra calories!

Step 4

You will probably lose the pounds faster than you get your tummy firm and tight again. Just hang in there and enjoy getting the exercise.

Ultimately, there are no true and total shortcuts. Celebrities may be able to get their bodies back post-pregnancy faster than you or I, but they probably spent the same number of total hours as either of us will.

I can tell you what each and every celebrity has to do to get a defined stomach again: Train the transverse abdominis and the pelvic floor! Whether they knew they were doing it or not, they had to in order to get a flat stomach again.

I do think it was a sexy move for Heidi Klum to get on that runway two months after having a baby. It sent the message that women can still be sexy after being pregnant. Just don't put that much pressure on yourself—it's not necessary; you'll get there. And make sure your partner knows it's not going to take two months . . . unless your partner wants to nanny, cook, and clean so you have time to work out and "not eat"!

Developing New Habits

One of the reasons losing weight is frequently so hard is because we all are creatures of habit. We develop routines and stick with them, even when they aren't really working for us. Your routine of eating extra calories is over unless you are breast-feeding. You can revisit that fun time when you get preggers again!

CHRISTINE, A MOTHER OF FIVE, TELLS US HOW YOU CAN GET IT DONE!

Being a mother has been one of the greatest joys and blessings in my life. My children are my life and I am so grateful to be a mother! It has also been a lesson in how to balance meeting others' needs as well as my own. There is much that we sacrifice as mothers. But I have found exercise to be both a sacrifice to make and a need to be met.

We have all heard, I am sure, about the physical benefits of exercise—basically a healthier body, inside and out. But exercise also has many spiritual, emotional, and mental benefits that help me as a mother. The last thing we may want to do, exhausted after being up all night with an infant, is exercise. However, I have found that energy begets energy. If I just put forth enough energy to take a walk, I find that I have the energy to complete the exercise session and actually have greater energy than if I hadn't exercised in the first place.

Having said all this, I will tell you how I find the means to exercise as a mother.

First, make it a priority. Put exercise on your list of important items to be done, or it won't get done. Find a time of the day that works best for you and have that be your time to do it. I find that if I don't get it done in the morning, I may not get it done. I am blessed with a supportive husband who can be home in the morning helping the children get ready for school, so I do an early-morning run on these days. On days that this doesn't work out, I am lucky to have a treadmill and a jogging stroller. I always have a backup plan if my initial plan can't happen. There will be bad-weather days or days when early morning just doesn't work out. Memberships to a community recreation center may be another option, or going with other mothers for some adult conversation. Keep trying things until you find something that works best for you.

Next, mental exertion. As the Nike slogan says, "Just do it!" Just as it takes stamina to exercise, it first takes the mental stamina to psych yourself into it. When I have those days that I am tempted to forgo exercise, I tell myself, "You'll feel better if you go." And I always do. It takes mental exertion to force yourself to go, but the exercise will release a lot of mental and physical tension and give you greater stamina.

Finally, stick with it! Don't give up. Exercise must be a habit, and it can be. Be patient in seeing results. You may feel completely worn out immediately after exercising. You may not drop a pound for a while. Even if you don't see the immediate results you want to see, you will notice gradual improvement in your general fitness. You may find that when your toddler throws a ball into the street you can actually run down the hill and catch it before it reaches the bottom. And you may also notice that you are not as winded as you make it back up the hill! Let these be huge accomplishments for you. Because they are!

If you can incorporate exercise into your life as a mother, both your physical and emotional health will benefit in order for you to carry out your responsibilities as a mother. It also sets an example that your children can follow. This is something that our children need to see and want to do for their own health benefits.

It is a challenge to find the means to exercise if you have children, but if I can do it, anyone can. And I must say that I have help because I pray for it. This is a real thing for me and it can be for you too.

May you make exercise a part of your life. And may you always be blessed by being a mother!

For me, three meals a day with two small snacks works well. These three meals are not large meals but are within a range of three hundred to four hundred calories. For some moms, five or six small meals a day works. My sister-in-law, on the other hand, goes from eating three meals a day when she's pregnant to two meals a day post-pregnancy. Now, while I don't recommend two meals a day, I do suggest you find a plan that works for you. The three-meals-a-day plan seems to occur in most families. If you are following this plan, try your best never to get to that ravenous point when your blood glucose drops and you eat anything and everything in sight. And, might I add, you *do not* need two dinners, one with the kids and one with your partner when the workday is done. It does not matter what time you consume the calories, but as always, no snacking after dinner!

By spreading out your calorie consumption throughout the day with five or six small meals (actually, we should call them tiny meals!), you avoid the peaks and valleys of hunger and get on a more level plane. As you adjust to mommyhood, or having four kids now, six mini-meals may be your best bet. Do what works for you, *but do not try both*—set your mind to either the three meals plus two snacks or the six minis.

Here's a sample day of ideal eating for weight loss if you aren't breast-feeding. A sound daily intake always includes protein, complex carbohydrates, fat, fiber, calcium, and water.

Breakfast: Fruit smoothie (made with yogurt)
Morning snack: String cheese and an apple
Lunch: Raspberry salad
Afternoon snack: Half of a small to medium-size baked potato with 2 percent melted cheese (or, if you must, less than 150 calories of candy)
Dinner: Flank steak fajitas

This book would be a thousand pages if it were up to me! But to keep it to a minimum, I encourage you to go to my Web site at momsintofitness.com/weight-loss-free-meal-plan to find the raspberry salad and flank steak fajitas recipes. You can print off a free one-week meal plan (which includes a how-to for breast-feeding with the meal plan), and at the same time you can calculate your metabolism and target weight (two things you will be doing in Part III). You can also find recipes at momsintofitness.com/recipes.

Now, if you are a person who loves meal plans, you will enjoy the seven-day sample menu at the back of the book or this free meal plan from my Web site. I am going to give you the tools in the 5-4-3-2-1 plan in Part III to make your own meal plan so you won't have to follow somebody else's for the rest of your life! If you need more of a boost, I also offer a sixty-day meal plan, which includes a fitness calendar and progress tracker.

And in Part III, when your life resumes some normalcy, we'll go over the 5-4-3-2-1 plan.

MAKE YOUR BODY
AN EFFICIENT FAT-BURNER

- It's not just your fitness regime that keeps you healthy. Your mind also needs to be healthy. So don't forget to go on a date with your partner, leave the kids at home with a sitter, and let loose!
- You don't want to cut nutrition when you cut calories. That being said, my motto is "You don't have to make the best choices, but the better choices!"
- It's OK to skip a meal every now and then—just don't make up for it late at night when your body wants to overindulge!
- Does your family eat out a lot? Make it a goal to eat only one meal a day out, not two or three. My husband eats lunch out every day, so I make dinner every night, since I know he didn't eat that healthy at lunch.
- Stay well hydrated. Water is considered a weight-loss aid and can also help improve your performance in daily tasks and exercise.
- Eat more fiber. Women should get at least twenty-five grams. Pregnant women should get twenty-five to thirty-five grams. Fiber keeps you full and flushes fat. Refer to page 45 in Part I for some easy ideas to add fiber!
- Continue taking omega-3 supplements after having your baby, especially if you are nursing.
- I had a friend once tell me to take 250 milligrams of magnesium with my multivitamin to keep my bowels regular. We all know the bowels take a while to get back to normal after pregnancy! Although I have not researched this and therefore don't recommend it.
- Most of all, sleep is important when trying to lose weight. I know you want to chuckle at the thought of more sleep right now, but if at all possible, grab your mom (or mother-in-law) for babysitting while you get some stuff done so you can hit the hay early tonight.
- Never cut all the fat from your diet. Doing this will make your body hold on to fat. Instead of cutting fat, make sure you eat the "right" fat. See page 48 for more on the "right" kinds of fat.

Don't Get Down

We all have to start somewhere. You may have never worked out and are starting at ground zero. Or you exercised throughout your pregnancy and are starting off a bit ahead of the game. Either way, the first several weeks after having a baby are going to feel like you're starting from *negative* ground zero. But if you worked out during pregnancy, you will vastly improve in minimal time. I will help you gradually bring your body back to the positive side!

Moderation, Not Deprivation

Just try it for the next several months—I promise it's the best "diet" you'll ever try! I don't expect you to go through life without little indulgences, like a glass of wine, a beer, or whatever you desire—the key is to drink one beer, not the six-pack. In fact, I have an indulgence of about 150 calories every day—either my Mr. Pibb with crushed ice or a handful of candy corn.

Order your chimichanga, but take half home. Enjoy a *snack-size* candy bar, not a *king-size* bar. Eat a serving of chips, *not the entire bag*. You get the picture. Get the body you desire by watching what you eat, not by finishing the bag before you realize you've overindulged again. And try to make the better choice 90 percent of the time, even if it isn't the best choice.

Finding a Balance

Find that balance not just in your life, but in your nutrition!

We're not going to dive into too many calculations, since you're on a time budget. Here's all you need to know about proteins, fats, and carbohydrates. The next and most important step in weight loss is staying within the calorie budget!

Carbohydrates: 40 to 60 percent
Fat: 20 to 30 percent
Protein: 10 to 20 percent

A typical meal is mostly made up of all three. For example, in a grilled cheese: the bread = carbs, the cheese = protein, and the olive oil and cheese = fat.

As you can see, my meal plans are not designed to get you to eat tofu and broccoli all the time. They are realistic in the sense that I am not trying to convert you to vegetarianism or even to get you to eat foods that you don't like. As I've said before, it's all about choosing better options and knowing that the best options are still out there and available if you choose to go that way.

> Look at the good, the bad, and the ugly. Check out my twelve-week challenge at lindsaybrin.com. You'll see pictures from the day I got home from the hospital and C-sections with both kids. Sometimes I cannot believe I posted all of my measurements and icky pictures, but here I am!

Staying Within Your Calorie Budget

METABOLISM

Metabolism is defined as the rate at which you burn calories. As I've said, toning exercises will boost your metabolism so you burn more calories at rest, or increase your basal metabolic rate (BMR). And this extra calorie burn helps get rid of stored fat. You will be boosting your metabolism with this fitness plan, so get ready to lose fat!

The formula for losing weight is quite simple: Either consume fewer calories than you need (your BMR calculation) or burn more calories than you consume. One is a nutrition-based approach; the other is exercise based. I want you to do both and maximize your time and effort to produce the kind of results you want. Also, be aware that most of us don't accurately estimate the number of calories we consume. Calculate your metabolism at momsintofitness.com/weight-loss-calculator.

EASY MEAL IDEAS

I know time is always at a premium, so here are a few ideas to help you plan your meals:

- **Breakfast:** Bars under two hundred calories; kids' bowl of fortified cereal with skim milk; low-fat yogurt with cereal or fruit mixed in; toasted English muffin with one tablespoon peanut butter.
- **Lunch:** Sandwich bread with fiber such as whole-wheat, bran, and sometimes multigrain. Or make it with a whole-wheat wrap. Add lean turkey, roast beef, or ham, and veggies such as tomato, red pepper, and cucumbers. Mustard is the best condiment calorie-wise. Add a half cup of soup for a filling lunch.
- **Dinner:** Use your grocery store for ready-made chicken, shrimp, and pork chops. Add half of a baked potato and one cup of veggies (I use the steam bags of frozen or fresh veggies) using the plate method described later on page 250. Of course, use smart condiments such as low-fat sour cream and extra virgin olive oil.
- Frozen TV dinners get a bad rap, but they are great for quick and healthy meals (although they usually contain a lot of sodium). Look for one around three hundred calories, with at least three grams of fiber and less than eight hundred milligrams of sodium. They are pretty easy to find these days. Just don't live on them! They can be a great snack as well, as long as they keep you within your calorie budget.

NUTRITION BARS ARE EASY AND QUICK. BUT ARE THEY HEALTHY?

With so many nutrition bars on the market, you really need to do your research before taking one down. A majority of them are about as nutritious as a candy bar—and have just as much sugar and fat. Do you really need all that protein? Not unless you're pregnant or breast-feeding. They are quick and make a great meal replacement, or you can have half as a snack. My favorites are the Luna Bar and Zone Perfect Bar; both are under two hundred calories. At the end of the day, as long as your snack calories fit into your overall daily allowance, the choice is up to you. There is no right or wrong answer on this; there are only different choices.

- **Snacks:** A small glass of milk and one small cookie; trail mix with cereal, raisins, and nuts; apple slices with peanut butter; baked potato with salt; cheese and crackers; shrimp cocktail; half of a sweet potato; four cups of light popcorn.

I hope you see by now that eating well doesn't have to mean eating bland or boring. No one can stick to any kind of nutritional plan if they hate what they are eating. I know one too many trainers who put their clients on the all-chicken-and-broccoli diet. In my mind that just sets you up for a crabby mood and an entire bag of chips and chocolate when you're off the diet. Again, it is all about making sensible choices and selecting the better of two options each time.

Breast-feeding, Exercise, and Nutrition

Whether or not a woman decides to breast-feed is a very personal choice. Since some women do choose to breast-feed, and their nutritional needs are different from women who don't, I feel the need to provide the information that follows. Plain and simple: Breast-feeding burns calories and you get to eat more! And for a majority of women, breast-feeding helps get them close to their pre-pregnancy weight and sometimes a few pounds under. But I have several very fit clients who, whether they breast-fed for three months or one year, were unable to shed the last five pounds to meet their target weight. Once they stopped breast-feeding, it was as if the weight just fell off. Whether it's fluid retention due to lack of periods while breast-feeding or your body's demand for additional fat in order to produce milk, the reality is that even if you breast-feed, you can experience difficulty in getting rid of those last few pounds.

If you are going to exercise (as you should) while breast-feeding, you do have to make some adjustments. Moderate aerobic activity has little effect on the quantity or quality of the milk your body produces or on the growth of your child. One study showed that high intensity exercise did increase the level of lactic acid that entered mother's milk, but the only real effect was on the taste of the milk, and some babies consumed slightly less as a result.[35] Lactic acid in your breast milk is not harmful; it probably just tastes different. So pump or express for two minutes before nursing, or used stored breast milk. Other studies show that the milk of nursing runners is no different from that of non-runners. Bottom line: It is perfectly safe to exercise and nurse your baby.

The Subcommittee on Nutrition During Lactation recommends consuming 1,500 to 1,800 calories *without* exercise. I usually consume 1,900 to 2,100 calories while I am breast-feeding, and if you're at all interested, I posted my food journal from my third week of breast-feeding on lindsaybrin.com. It's far from perfect, but it's honest. Click on Breastfeeding Weight Loss.

> You can feel your stomach shrinking as you breast-feed! Oxytocin is released, which causes your uterus to contract—you literally feel your stomach shrinking. Always activate your core when nursing.

My advice is to basically follow the nutrition regimen you followed during your pregnancy. Babies get what they need from breast milk at the mother's expense, just like they got what they needed while they were in your belly. So make sure to continue your prenatal vitamins, omega-3s, and iron pills (if you were anemic during pregnancy you may want to ask your doctor if you still need them).

If you are breast-feeding you are going to have higher calorie needs than those who are not. Breast-feeding has many benefits for both you and your child, aiding in the physical, emotional, and practical needs of you both. Women who breast-feed have been found to return to their pre-pregnancy weight more quickly and the uterus returns to its normal size more rapidly.

> ACOG recommends drinking according to thirst. But remember when you are exercising you need to replenish that water. So I recommend drinking eight to sixteen ounces every fifteen to twenty-five minutes during vigorous exercise, and sometimes more with breast-feeding.

Your body requires an extra 330 calories a day during breast feeding.[36] While your calorie needs are higher you should still aim to incorporate nutritious foods that fit into the appropriate balance, variety, and moderation.

But this is not one size fits all—you must monitor your caloric intake and decide whether your body needs two hundred or five hundred extra calories. If you are losing more than a pound a week, you probably need closer to five hundred.

Rule #8: Calorie counting during breast-feeding is difficult; monitor weight loss by watching the scale.

ON THAT NOTE

Some research suggests 500 extra calories, instead of the 330 mentioned above. I suggest you speak with your doctor and monitor your weight loss. Keep it between one half and one pound per week. At the same time you must make sure your baby is getting enough milk. Also make sure your extra calories come from protein—you need more now than you did during pregnancy!

Healthy fats (DHA) can be transferred to infants only if Mom is receiving adequate amounts.[37] All the more reason to concentrate on good fats. Seafood is one of the biggest contributors of DHA.

Healthy women can continue to exercise without it interfering with the quantity or quality of breast milk. But make sure to consume even more liquids, and more calories. If your baby is fussy when fed within sixty minutes after you exercise, you may need to change your exercise time.

Since breast-feeding increases your needs for fat and protein, you may notice you hold on to an extra five or ten pounds. All that means is you don't have much fat to spare!

The new mom's shortcut to weight loss:

At four weeks postpartum try to add one of the following tricks to your current eating habits.

Week 4: Add one glass of water before eating a meal.

Week 5: Add a piece of fruit to breakfast.

Week 6: Add a vegetable to dinner.

Week 7: Replace sugar snacks with high-volume snacks that contain a carbohydrate and a protein, such as a banana with one tablespoon of peanut butter or crackers with 2 percent cheese.

Week 8: Cut portions by 20 percent (see box "Why 20 Percent?") unless you are breast-feeding.

Week 9: Notice the difference between head hunger and real hunger. Are you hungry because you saw a commercial for a tasty food, or does your body really need energy?

Week 10: Add some calcium.

Week 11: Add a vegetable to lunch.

- If you are not breast-feeding, week eight is a good time to look at the nutrition plan in Part III. It's a little more strict and will help you lose faster.

Week 12: Make your main dish vegetables, instead of meat. Americans overeat protein by 200 percent. Keep in mind protein is found in nuts, beans, dairy, and eggs. Vegetables will fill you up with fewer calories.

Week 13: Eat high-volume foods, not "empty" foods. High-volume foods include fiber and water to keep you satisfied, and they provide numerous nutrients and vitamins. Examples include vegetables, fruit, soups, whole-grain items, and nuts. See page 295 for high-volume recipes.

Week 14: Learn to prepare healthy meals ahead of time!

WHY 20 PERCENT?

A registered dietitian once told me we don't notice if 20 percent of our usual food intake is missing, but we may notice 30 percent. So get rid of 20 percent of the calories on your plate. And this doesn't mean get rid of veggies—veggies are low in calories and high in fiber and water, which keeps you full.

Dining Out

Here are some rules for dining out. Don't forget there is a list of "better" fast-food choices in the pregnancy section, on page 64.

Dining Out Rules

- Choose clear broth soups such as chicken noodle or minestrone to fill you up.
- Start with a small side salad (dressing on the side).
- Package half of your plate to go.
- A meal can be made up of side items such as a side salad, a baked potato, vegetables, beans, pilafs, shrimp cocktail, soup, and so on.
- When ordering meat, fish, or poultry, make sure it's steamed, baked, grilled, broiled, roasted, or poached. No fried meat!
- Avoid the words *creamy, cheesy, breaded, batter-dipped*.
- Avoid casseroles and gravy (or heavy sauce).
- Have tea or coffee for dessert.
- No buffets.
- Forget jumbo, large, supersize, etc.

Eating for Weight Loss

If you are breast-feeding, you should add a few hundred calories.

Breakfast (about 300–400 calories)

- ½ whole-wheat bagel with reduced-fat peanut butter
- ½ English muffin with turkey bacon and 1 egg (or substitute)
- Oatmeal and 1 apple
- 1 cup high-fiber cereal with 1 cup skim milk
- 1 banana with 2 tablespoons peanut butter

Check out our easy breakfast recipes at momsintofitness.com.

Lunch (about 300–400 calories)

- Out to lunch? Take half home for tomorrow.
- Grilled chicken sandwich and small salad.
- Low-sodium soup and crackers.
- Whole-wheat pita with chicken, tuna, or turkey, cucumbers, tomatoes, lettuce, and peppers with light dressing or mustard.
- Salad with light dressing (light on the cheese, eggs, and bacon; protein is calorie dense).

2 Snacks (about 150–300 calories each)

- Shrimp cocktail
- Low-fat yogurt with sprinkles or crunchy cereal
- 100-calorie pudding with strawberries to dip
- Plain baked potato with skin
- Small salad
- Air-popped popcorn (try the popcorn seasoning in the spice aisle)
- Veggies and hummus
- 1 cup fruit
- ½ protein bar
- Other half of English muffin from breakfast with 1 tablespoon peanut butter

Small Dinner (about 300–400 calories)

- Grilled salmon (pregnant women should avoid wild salmon), asparagus, and ½ baked potato
- Black beans and rice, served with a veggie
- Grilled chicken on a salad
- Pan-grilled quesadilla: whole-wheat tortilla with grilled chicken, skim-milk cheese, and veggies
- Pork chop, brown rice, and small salad
- Stir-fry: 2 teaspoons olive oil, any lean meat, peppers, tomatoes, green beans, squash, or any vegetables you like. Serve over ½ cup brown rice.
- 1 low-fat frozen dinner with a side of veggies

We'll talk more about nutrition in Part III, but for now, the important thing is to bond with your baby—remember, every time you pick up your newborn you should engage your PF and TA—and spend as much time as possible healing and taking care of yourself. You deserve that kind of a break, and eating well is just another way you can better take care of yourself!

· 9 ·

GETTING YOUR BODY BACK

Getting to the Core Issues

everal years ago, long before I was pregnant with my first child, my husband and I were invited to dinner at a friend's house. Our hostess, Kelly, had also invited her mother and her sister Sarah. Sarah was several months pregnant and was joined by her husband, Randy. Before dinner, we were seated in the living room talking about kids and pregnancy issues, all of us very excited for the proud mother-to-be. When we were seated at the dining room table, Randy asked his mother-in-law, "Virginia, what was it like giving birth to Sarah?"

At that point Kelly came out of the kitchen with a large turkey on a serving platter. We all oohed and ahhed. Kelly's mom, an attractive woman in her mid-fifties, attired in a very tasteful Dior suit, pointed at the main course and said, "Imagine squeezing that out of your penis."

"Mother!" Sarah and Kelly squealed in unison.

Virginia took a sip of her wine and set it down, nodding at Randy. "He asked."

Not about to be outdone, Randy said, "Well, if it was frozen it wouldn't be so bad."

Virginia wagged her index finger at him. "No, no, my dear. Not frozen. Not cooked. A live turkey and one in the mood to peck and claw."

My husband and I looked at each other, trying to stifle both a laugh and a horrified gasp. Randy mumbled something about mashed potatoes, and the conversation resumed a more normal tone and content.

I don't know if you think Virginia's description is accurate or not, but by this time you're at least a better judge than you were pre-delivery. All I know is that I could not get that image out of my mind. I found it funny that Kelly's mom had been able to come up with such a graphic comparison for her son-in-law. Fortunately, despite that lingering image, when I was pregnant I never had bad turkey birthing dreams! Sure, like most moms-to-be, I had a lot of anxiety associated with what labor might be like. Few of us enjoy pain, and the first time you're pregnant, you are entering into unknown territory. You can read all the books, talk to friends and family, but this is one of those you-gotta-do-it-to-understand-it situations. For me, having a C-section instead of a vaginal delivery was determined at thirty-six weeks, when Taylor was still lying sideways. And in my mind, if you have a healthy baby, that's giving birth, whether you squeezed the turkey out or didn't feel a thing.

Life After Baby

The great thing about finally delivering a baby is that a lot of those doubts and insecurities about labor go away instantly. Talk about your life-altering, life-affirming, life-loving moments! I was on such a high. Yeah, having to be sutured—I asked for stitches or tape and not staples—meant that I couldn't watch the first baths. I did feel a little bit like saying, "Hey, over here! I did all the hard work for the past nine months—can I get a little attention?" but that only lasted for a second or two. I knew that the focus in my life and my husband's life had now changed. We were baby centered. I like that term because while our lives did revolve around our infant and her needs, we weren't baby obsessed. *Centered* means that we had a point of balance around which other things revolved, but there were still other things in our lives.

Vision Board

Goal setting and motivation are always important. Get a cheap bulletin board next time you're at the store. Now pin up three goals. That can be your swimsuit, a picture of you at your best, and a "stay away from the fridge" sign. That's what I had pinned up on mine, and I cringed for the first six weeks as I looked at my calendar swimsuit shot from when I was an NFL cheerleader. But once it was time to stop breast-feeding, I needed some extra motivation to turn off my pregnancy and breast-feeding extra calorie consumption.

One of the best pieces of advice I got was from the nurse practitioner I worked with in a pilot study on exercise, pregnancy, and postpartum depression. She said it's so important for parents to prepare ahead of time for life after baby. The tendency is to focus so intently on the pregnancy and labor that when the baby arrives parents go into a bit of a panic. They don't think about how each of their roles is going to be changed. If they don't prepare in advance, a big fat fight can arise. My husband and I had talked a lot about what the addition to our family was going to do in terms of assigning us different responsibilities. We each had careers and ran our own businesses. Maybe because when we got married we had to talk about how his busy dental practice and my busy fitness company were going to be able to thrive and eventually expand, we were used to having those kinds of conversations. I'm a very orderly and precise person, which can make my husband crazy at times, and I need to know and be able to develop all kinds of action plans in advance of certain events to be in my comfort zone. Dividing up household chores and developing a schedule that would allow each of us to continue our careers and spend time with our precious new child was extremely important.

Help

Yes, I know that *help* is a four-letter word, but it is one that as a new mom you need to be able to speak with clarity and precision. There is so much pressure on us as women and mothers to be the perfect mom; the know-it-all, do-it-all mother image is an enormous burden that's placed on us and that we sometimes place on ourselves. We all want to do it all, but doing it all should include being able to delegate and ask for assistance. There is no shame in having family or friends come in to help you post-pregnancy. Hiring a nanny, full-time or part-time, doesn't mean that you care any less about your child. Yes, we all want to put our children's needs ahead of our own, but that doesn't mean that our kids are the only ones who have needs. Take people up on their offers to come and watch the baby for an hour so that you can get your exercise, take a walk outside to clear your head, or nap. Being able to ask for help is a sign of strength and confidence in your own ability. It is not a sign of weakness or failure!

Finding the Time to Exercise

Obviously, postpartum exercise is important, and finding time to do it is likely to be more difficult than it was pre–labor and delivery. In fact, as I've already mentioned. I don't really want you to think about exercise for the first four weeks. You will do a few simple movements that take five minutes, tops, every other day. And most likely, unless you truly are Supermom, there will be days you are so stressed out that all you want to do is take a nap and forget your ever-growing to-do list. And some days that's just what you should do! But remember, asking for help and a half hour to an hour a day a few times a week to work on your body is not a bad thing. You deserve to be healthy and fit, and you can do all the things you want to do for your family only if you are those two things.

At the beginning, just after childbirth, the kinds of exercise you will be able to do will require minimal time. In fact, two days after a vaginal birth, you will begin doing Kegel exercises and engaging your TA muscles. You can do these at any time during the day, and they don't require you to put on your workout gear. I'll review those exercises and introduce new ones in the next chapter. Keep in mind that every woman will respond differently to childbirth. If you don't feel ready to move beyond the Kegel and TA exercises, then you shouldn't push it. Here are the four phases of your initial core exercise routine:

Phase 1 (weeks 0–6): Reestablish
Phase 2 (weeks 6–8): Recover and retrain
Phase 3 (weeks 9–11): Condition
Phase 4 (weeks 12–14): Shrink

In these four phases, the goal is to train the pelvic floor and deep abdominal wall, to tone the core from the inside out. For most moms the initial desire is to get rid of the "mom pooch" as soon as possible. After nine months of watching your waistline first expand and then disappear, you're excited to see how after giving birth that bubble has gone away. My mom always told me she walked out of the hospital in her jeans. Yeah, right! I walked out in my maternity pants, but by the next week all I had left was a small but stubborn bit of excess that I really wanted to get rid of.

More than likely your stomach muscles will not return to "normal" unless a concentrated exercise effort is made.

The CFS Method

The reason many women believe that the mom pooch is a stubborn pooch that won't lie down or go away when you want it to is that they don't work from the inside out. Traditional abdominal workouts can actually push your muscles out, increasing your waistline—exactly what you don't want to happen. You're building and strengthening them, but by making them larger and forcing them out, you're actually making them more prominent and noticeable. That's why I created what I call the CFS method. CFS stands for Core Firing Sequence. By firing (using) those deep, innermost muscles first, you will be able to have the flat stomach we all desire.

If you were doing the workouts in Part I, good for you. You'll probably get that flat stomach sooner than someone who is picking up this book post-pregnancy. But for those of you who didn't do those exercises, don't worry. You will get there! It may just take a bit longer, but the time and effort will be worth it. And the exercises you will be doing will be easy and efficient. None of that five-hundred-crunches-a-day nonsense!

WHY THE CORE AND WHY CFS?

One of the reasons you need to add the CFS exercises to any other workout routine you may be doing is that after pregnancy, your uterus shrinks about a finger width every day. In five to six weeks, it will return to pre-pregnancy size. That means in that time it will go from the size of a watermelon to the size of an orange. Pretty impressive, right? Your body is remarkably adaptable, and your recovery to pre-pregnancy hormone levels, uterus size, and so on is a postpartum miracle. Your core muscles are just as adaptable. Your body is a machine in the several weeks following birth. But you do need to help that miracle along.

BEGIN

In Phase 1 of the CFS routine, you will start by finding and then training your pelvic floor. The pelvic floor is the foundation and the bottom of your core—think of a sling running from front to back. Your abs cannot function without it. You will see a number of exercises that include rotation, balance, and stabilization. This variety, combined with the use of the pelvic floor and transverse abdominis, is the basis of the CFS method. You will begin pelvic floor exercises within two days of a normal vaginal delivery. The ab work will begin about six weeks later, once you have your doctor's permission. This method will not only help you look good; it will help you do functional things without pain. You can get down on the floor and play with baby, jump without peeing, and lift baby pain-free.

Working Your Core, Revisited

Your core is essentially the center of your body—more specifically, your abdominal muscles and the muscles of the hips, butt, back, and pelvic floor. All of your core muscles work together as a unit; they are all connected by fascia, a band of connective tissue.

We reviewed core activation in Part I; please refer to page 92 to refresh yourself. Or if you just picked up the book, read Chapter 4. Your muscles have the same action and reaction during and after pregnancy, so it's important you understand how they work in your quest for a flat stomach.

The Core's "Fifth" Muscle

It's not really a muscle, but it functions like a muscle would. It's called your fascia. And if you recall, we talked about it in Part I. Within six weeks of delivery, your fascia is back to 90 percent of its strength and will help compact your stomach, along with your PF and TA.

Find Your Pelvic Floor

It's so important! You can find these moves on page 82.

Remember, doing Kegels during and after pregnancy will help urinary incontinence when jumping, sneezing, and coughing!

Find Your TA and Keep It Activated!

Core activation: While sitting or standing, place one hand across your lower abdomen, just below your belly button. Draw your abdominals away from your hand so you can see light between your hand and your stomach. Breathe normally—this is the tricky part. You need to learn the difference between activating the TA and sucking it in.

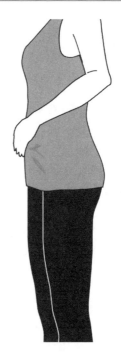

Posture and Balance

You don't need to set aside time to activate your TA while sitting or standing. Whenever you are holding your baby, it is so important to do this exercise to help support your spine and maintain proper posture. You can always activate the TA while holding your baby; it just takes a little concentration. Instead of letting the abs hang out while holding the baby, draw them away from the baby. You should also focus on holding up your pelvic floor and holding in your transverse while driving, talking on the phone, and, of course, exercising!

Stretching Is Equally Important

Along with doing locating and strengthening exercises for the abdominals and pelvic floor, it is important that you stretch. The tendency for all your muscles when stressed (and they are during pregnancy and child birth) is for them to contract. In the three phases after the initial recovery phase you will be doing a series of stretches concentrating on the back of your body. Your hamstrings and lower back, as well as the muscles of your chest, really tighten up during pregnancy. And yes, sometimes the last thing you want to do is stretch—but you cannot drop this important component. You have a million other things to do, but take five minutes to find your Zen and lengthen your muscles.

You will notice that you stretch your hips and quadriceps before doing all ab exercises. After pregnancy your core is weaker—usually weaker than your quadriceps and hips. These stronger muscles will take over and you will end up using your legs instead of your abs. So stretch your legs before core work to keep them from contracting.

POST-PREGNANCY STRETCHES

1. Knees in: Lie on your back with your legs extended in front you, your heels touching, your toes pointing slightly out to the side, and your arms at your side. Raise your knees toward your chest and bring your hands to your knees. Gently pull your knees closer to your chest. Be sure to keep your spine aligned and try to keep your lower back on the floor. Advanced modification: As you hold your knees, straighten your legs, and hold for 20 seconds.

2. Lying spinal twist: Lie on your back with your arms extended out from your shoulders (your body should form a *T*). Raise your right knee up toward your chest and then out toward your left arm. Lower and repeat on the other side. Again, try to keep your spine aligned and in contact with the floor. Advanced modification: Extend your right leg after raising your knee toward your opposite arm and hold for 20 seconds.

3. Downward dog:

   - Lower yourself to the floor so that you're on your hands and knees with wrists beneath your shoulders and knees below your hips.
   - Curl your toes under and push yourself back with your arms while raising your hips and straightening your legs.
   - Let your head hang. Prevent yourself from scrunching your shoulders around your ears by moving your shoulder blades away, toward your hips.
   - Hold for 20 seconds.

4. Walk back: From the downward dog, walk your hands toward your feet until all your weight is on your feet and you can lift your hands off the floor. Bend forward and try to touch either your knees, shins, or toes, depending on your flexibility, and hold for 20 seconds.

5. Single-leg cross staff: Sit down with both legs extended in front of you. Draw one heel up toward your crotch and place your foot inside the

knee or thigh of the extended leg so that your legs form the number four. Sit as straight as possible, and bring your head and chest out over your straight leg, reaching for your foot and slowly lowering as far as you can. Return to starting position, switch legs, and repeat, holding each side for 20 seconds.

6. Chest stretch: Place the palm of your right hand on a wall and turn your torso to your left and away from the wall, opening up the chest.

Stretching is a wonderful time for baby tummy time. More exercises with baby to come in Chapter 11.

Diastasis Recti Remedy

Please see page 84 for how you can self-evaluate for this condition. If you have diastasis recti, you must do each of the exercises below before beginning Phase 1. Once you have mastered these, you can move to Phase 1, which can take anywhere from one to several weeks to master, depending on the severity of your diastasis. For each exercise, you will do 1 set of 10 or as many as you can without pain.

1. Back press: Stand with your back against a wall, your feet comfortably apart, and your hands at your sides. While engaging your PF and TA, raise one arm over your head as you bend into a shallow squat. Switch arms while staying in the shallow squat. Remember: Engage your PF and TA while doing this exercise! Refer to page 216 for an illustration.
2. The cough: With a towel on your stomach to add pressure, either lie down or sit, making sure that your knees are bent. While engaging your PF and TA, cough.
3. Assisted crunch: Lie on the floor with your knees raised and your heels approximately eighteen inches from your butt. Place a rolled towel under the center of your back. Grab each end of the towel, and use your arms to help you perform a crunch by crisscrossing the towel and assisting yourself in the upward portion of the crunch.
4. Opposites: Sit on a chair or exercise ball. Hold the left side of your stomach with your right hand and lean back to your right, with your right arm reaching twelve to eighteen inches behind you.

5. Pelvic rotations: Stand with your feet comfortably apart and your baby in your arms. Keep your knees soft. Without turning your feet or your knees, rotate from your hips to the left, back to center, and then to the right. If you are rotating more than just a couple of inches, you know you are twisting your legs.

Note: It's important to make sure you do not have a hernia; otherwise you should be able to create a healthy core again, even if you have diastasis.

PELVIC TILTS

Pelvic tilts are an excellent core exercise and help relieve lower-back pain.

1. Lie on your back with the crook of your knees bent over a couch. There will be a space between the floor and your lower back, as well as your neck. This is because your core is not activated yet.
2. Inhale, and as you exhale, tilt your pelvis toward your belly button. It is a small move and you won't really see much movement in your tummy. Continue to pull without letting your stomach "pooch out."
3. Release.
4. Remember to use your core, not your buttocks or thighs. If you feel your lower body contracting, release completely and try again.

How Do I Deal with Urinary Incontinence?

If you were to believe the commercials for things like Depend undergarments, you might think urinary incontinence afflicts only older women. That is a myth. Fifty-three percent of women experience it after their first pregnancy. And 85 percent experience it after subsequent pregnancies. Sixty to 80 percent of women injure nerve endings during birth, which damages pelvic floor muscles and affects the ability to control the bladder and sphincter. A midline episiotomy, especially fourth degree (first being smallest), can create dysfunction of the pelvic floor, which also interrupts core function (remember, the pelvic floor is part of your core).[38] Several of the tools and instruments that doctors use to assist you in giving birth, including vacuums and forceps, can cause PF dysfunction. Women who have had C-sections tend to have less trauma to these muscles, but incontinence is still present from the baby sitting on the bladder during pregnancy (your uterus is on top of your bladder).

A study published in the *American Journal of Obstetrics and Gynecology* found that moms who'd had a C-section were less likely to do pelvic floor exercises, probably because they didn't push the baby through the pelvic floor. However, it's pregnancy itself that affects the pelvic floor. Moms who have vaginal births with deep tears will have more damage to the pelvic floor.

There are two ways to help urinary incontinence before considering surgery: bladder training and pelvic floor exercises. Before we begin those exercises, let's determine if you have the problem:

Are you incontinent?[39]

Do you use the restroom every two to four hours?
Do you use the restroom at least once during the night?
Do you have normal urges (i.e., you're not running to the restroom with urine trickling down your leg)?

There are hormonal stages throughout your cycle than can affect your answers to these questions. But most of the time your answers should be yes for normal bladder function. If you have to go more frequently, get up at night more often, and if you have sudden painful urges, then chances are you have an incontinence issue. Remember that caffeine is a bladder stimulant, so you might want to stop drinking as much or remove it from your diet entirely while training your pelvic floor.

If you do the PF identification and Kegel exercises, you will be doing exactly what you need to do to work on incontinence issues. Incontinence can be brought on by stresses to your system; for example, when you laugh, cough, or sneeze. The "squeeze before you sneeze method"—activating the muscles of the PF before letting go with your sneeze—is an effective means of stopping leaks. Exercise can also lead to incontinence, particularly higher-impact activities such as step exercises.

Before you consider surgical options or costly medications, be sure to try these interventions. If you are using the correct muscles when doing the Kegel exercises and the various PF exercises, then chances are you can avoid those more drastic measures. By the time you build up to doing fifty to a hundred Kegels per day, you will most likely have experienced improvement.

There are also other things you can do to help with incontinence. Training your bladder can be as simple as scheduling a bathroom break every two hours. Every other day, add thirty minutes to that time. Your goal is to be able to last two to four hours between visits. To do this, you can use two techniques: bracing and distraction. The first involves engaging those PF muscles when you feel the urge to go. After holding for ten seconds, release. Distraction is as simple as the name implies. Find other things to think about and do instead of heading to the bathroom. When your mind and body are actively engaged, you tend to be able to last longer. A more serious training technique involves biofeedback. Only a doctor can work with you using this technique, which involves placing an electrode in the vagina. The electrode measures the intensity and duration of your Kegel contractions and helps you to gauge better how effectively you are squeezing.

Some women also lack control of their bowel movements; these exercises will help with that as well. A more serious difficulty can develop, however. In the most serious cases of damage to the muscles of the pelvic floor, your muscles could prolapse. Pelvic organ prolapse occurs when the pelvic floor muscles become weak or damaged and can no longer support the pelvic organs. The uterus is the only organ that actually falls into the vagina. When the bladder and bowel slip out of place, they push up against the walls of the vagina. While prolapse is not considered a life-threatening condition, it may cause a great deal of discomfort and distress.

One of my friends had a level four episiotomy. I had no idea what a level four entailed until she told me she was cut from front to back, literally. She is going to have a harder time with incontinence than my cousin, who had one stitch. And both my cousin and friend will have to work harder on their incontinence than I did. There are pros and cons with both vaginal and C-section deliveries!

Phase 1: Reestablish (Weeks 0–6)

Phase 1 is perhaps the most important part of the program. You will either be finding for the first time or, if you worked out during pregnancy, reconnecting with your pelvic floor. I call this the Core Firing Sequence, because you want to engage these specific muscles in the right order. Think of this as a kind of rocket firing countdown. Each step transitions into the next. You will always begin with firing the first of the muscles—those in your pelvic floor. Eventually, this will become an automatic, subconscious response. You will end up doing it all day, creating that flat tummy!

If You Had Your Child Three Years Ago and Are Just Starting Out

You will be able to move through phases 2 and 3 a lot quicker, but you still need to spend time in Phase 1 to train your core. Although for your cardio, since your body is not healing, you can use the cardio portions in Phase 3 or 4 (whichever you're comfortable with).

If you've ever been in physical therapy, you know you have to use a lot of your subconscious. When I was in PT after an ACL tear I had to re-teach my leg muscles what they were supposed to do; they kind of forgot. When you walk, you don't think of all the various movements your leg and foot muscles (as well as other parts of your body) go through to keep you going, particularly when you aren't walking on a level surface. You don't have to think about it; you just do it.

In this phase you should not do any core exercises, just some PF movements. Your body's energy needs to go to healing. If you notice your energy is zapped, it's not just because you have a newborn waking you up at night, but because your body's energy is going toward healing. Think about it as moving the furniture back—everything was arranged differently during pregnancy. You cannot control the inside healing, so be patient and listen to your body. Do not exercise too early. as your bladder, among other things, isn't back to normal yet and stress can cause incontinence.

Make sure you read each description in depth and understand each movement before beginning the exercises. We're going away from traditional abdominal work and crunches to wake up the pelvic floor and TA! The moves are less intense and obvious, so for the pelvic floor you are going to stimulate muscles you won't necessarily feel all the time. Sometimes it can take several months for this "subconsciousness" to kick in on the pelvic floor. You are also going to be reestablishing the blood flow and oxygen flow to all of your muscles. Your body is used to supporting your uterus and baby with oxygen and blood flow, so restoring pre-pregnancy function is all a part of Phase 1.

Phases 1 through 4 will last from zero to fourteen weeks, depending upon how you feel and how frequently you are able to work out during this time. I know that you are extremely busy, so I suggest that you work out three times per week, or every other day. Now is the time to ease back into your workouts and try to incorporate them into your new schedule. The more work you are able to do now, the sooner you will move on, but you are not in a race. You will get back to that target weight you set for yourself. Remember that vision board, your photographs, and that outfit you want to get into? Now is the time to do as much mental preparation as physical work.

PHASE 1

Exercise	Sets x Reps/Frequency	How To
Core activation	1 x 10 M W F	While sitting or standing, place one hand across your lower abdomen, just below your belly button. Draw your abdominals away from your hand so you can see light between your hand and stomach. Breathe normally.
Pelvic floor warm-up	1 x 10 M W F	Lie on the floor with your knees bent or your feet on the couch or the floor. Place one hand on your belly. Perform a Kegel. When you feel strong enough and pain-free enough, add a small pelvic tilt after each Kegel. (Go to page 210 for the sidebar on pelvic tilts.) See figure on page 215.
Kegels	3 x 10 M W F	Refer to page 82 for description.

Exercise	Sets x Reps/Frequency	How To
Back press	5 x 10 seconds M W F	Stand with your back against a wall, your feet comfortably apart, and your hands at your sides. While engaging your PF and TA, raise one arm over your head as you bend into a shallow squat. Bring your arm down as you return to the starting position. Switch arms and repeat. See figures on page 216.
Cardio only: Leisure walking	Try to incorporate 10–20 minutes every other day, if not every day. Break when needed.	

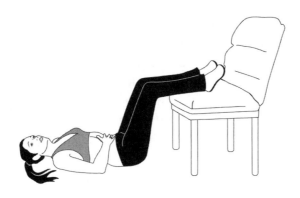

Pelvic floor warm-up

If you're not used to having boobs (like me), don't forget to wear a very supportive bra when exercising!

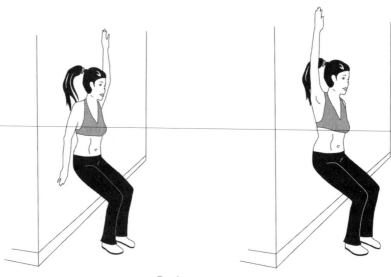

Back press

THE "SHELF" AFTER A C-SECTION

Many clients I have worked with complain about the shelf that protrudes over their C-section scar. So I went straight to the source—the man who performed my first C-section. The good news: You can and will get rid of it if you make your muscles work! Dr. Kent Snowden told me the shelf is most likely fatty tissue damage. And after all the swelling goes down and you are back to normal (maybe six months down the line), all you should be left with is scar tissue.

I requested stitches instead of staples. But the good ol' doc told me the end result is the same, although he likes to take his time and stitch his patients up.

Phase 2: Recover and Retrain (Weeks 6–8)

Once you've reached weeks six to eight postpartum and you've been consistently completing the movements in Phase 1, it's time to transition to the next phase. This timetable is for women who have given birth to a single child either vaginally or through C-section, with no complications. For some C-sections and twins (vaginal or C-section), wait until you are eight to ten weeks out from labor before beginning Phase 2. You will need that additional time to heal. You can also use this program if it has been years since you gave birth. Spend two weeks doing the exercises in the following table and add in two days of cardio workouts. Again, make sure you have your doctor's permission.

This is the most difficult phase, since you're going to establish that subconscious connection and make using your PF and TA a habit. You will not necessarily feel the burn in these exercises, but it's important you don't concentrate on traditional abdominal training at this point. Now is when you need to make the commitment to finding the time for working out. You and your baby probably don't have a consistent schedule yet, but hopefully you're getting more sleep at this point. This is your chance to establish the routine that will carry you through meeting your post-pregnancy goals and beyond. A month after giving birth, I know that I was feeling a lot better, and I hope you will be also!

> I've listed repetitions for you, but cannot emphasize enough paying attention to your own comfort level. You know your body better than anyone—heck you had a baby—and your body is intelligent enough to tell you when you're doing too much.

At this point you are ready to move into my *Core Firing Sequence Method* and *Postnatal Boot Camp* DVDs, if you'd like to incorporate them. You can find them on momsintofitness.com. Follow Phase 2 for the CFS method (if you have diastasis recti, follow Phase 1) and follow the twelve-week program on *Postnatal Boot Camp*. All of my workouts, whether in this book or on my DVDs, are quick and efficient—twenty-five minutes, tops!

PHASE 2

Exercise	Sets x Reps/Frequency	How To
Runner's lunge	Hold 20 seconds each leg. M W F	Take a step forward with one foot, bend the trailing leg so that your knee touches the floor, and place your hands on the floor. You should feel the stretch in your hip flexors and quads. See figure on page 222.

Exercise	Sets x Reps/Frequency	How To
Core activation	1 x 10 M W F	Same as Phase 1.
Pelvic floor warm-up	1 x 10 M W F	Same as Phase 1.
Hip slings	1 x 20 M W F	From the pelvic floor warm-up position, keep your belly button drawn toward your back. Now pull one hip closer to the bottom of your rib cage, as if you are pinching your love handles. Do not squeeze your butt.
Pelvic tilt with march	Beginners: 2 x 10 Veterans: 3 x 10 M W F	From the pelvic floor warm-up position, place your hands under your hips. Slowly bring one knee toward your chest without letting the knee bend any more, keeping the PF and TA engaged and your back on the floor. Switch. See figures on page 221.
Hand crunch	Beginners: 1 x 25 Veterans: 2 x 20 M W F	Begin in crunch position with one hand on your belly. Crunch up, making sure your stomach does not pooch out—but keep your PF and TA activated so your stomach stays flat. Your hand is on your belly to feel if you pooch out.
Modified boomerang	1 x 20 M W F	Lie on your stomach and place your elbows on the floor directly under your shoulders with your legs extended. Raise yourself so that your body is supported by your knees and elbows. Pull your navel in so you maintain a straight line from the top of your head to your knees. Hold this position. Rotate and drop one hip toward the floor, then the other. See figures on page 222.

Exercise	Sets x Reps/Frequency	How To
Half seal	Work up to 2 x 10 by week 8 M W F	Lie on your stomach and place your hands under your shoulders with your fingers closed. Lock your feet together with the tops touching the floor. Inhale, and as you exhale peel your upper body off the floor. Your hands are there only for balance—do not push yourself up; use your back muscles. If you had a C-section, make sure lying on your stomach does not hurt your incision. See figure on page 222.
Bridge	Beginners: 1 x 30 seconds Veterans: 2 x 30 seconds M W F	Lie on your back with your knees bent, palms facedown at your side, and feet shoulder-width apart. Lift your hips off the floor and hold. See figure on page 222.
Couch squat	Beginners: 2 x 10 Veterans: 2 x 20 M W F	Stand in front of a couch with your arms extended in front of you and your palms down, feet shoulder-width apart. Bend your knees so that you almost touch the cushion with your butt. Keep your knees behind your toes and your abdominals in. Veterans: Hold a 3–8-pound weight with both hands. See figure on page 222.
Modified push-ups	Beginners: 3 x 5 Veterans: 2 x 15 M W F	Use a couch or a stair and with your knees on the floor and your hands on the object, do a push-up.*

*If your wrists bother you as you are doing push-ups, you may need to do some exercises for carpal tunnel (remember, carpal tunnel can happen during pregnancy). Holding a 1- to 3-pound weight, place your wrist on the edge of a table so your hand is over the edge. Lift and lower your fist about 10 times, then flip your palm over and repeat.

Exercise	Sets x Reps/Frequency	How To
Stationary lunge	Beginners: 2 x 10 each leg Veterans: 2 x 20 each leg M W F	Place one foot in front of you and one foot behind you, about three feet apart. Stay upright, but bend both knees almost to ninety degrees. Straighten your legs and repeat. See figure on page 222.
Cardio block	M W F Try to finish 15–20 reps within 1 minute. Beginners: 1 set Veterans: 2 sets	1 minute of each: *Quarter speed squats:* Perform squat, lowering only a quarter of the way down to keep quick pace. *Touchdowns:* Stand with feet two feet apart, run in place by lifting knees four times. Touch the ground with one hand. *Lateral ski:* Stand with feet two feet apart, shifting weight to one leg as you hop from side to side. *Side squats:* Stand with feet shoulder-width apart. Step to one side and perform squat. Return to center position and switch sides. *Mountain climbers:* From plank position, "run" your knees in and out. Every time your right knee comes in, it counts as one set.
Cardio only: If you're unable to go outside or use a treadmill, do 2–3 sets of the cardio block.	T or Th	20-minute speed walk. Veterans: Add 1 minute of jogging every 3 or 4 minutes.
Kegels	3 x 10 at bedtime	See page 82 for description.

Exercise	Sets x Reps/Frequency	How To
Pelvic rotations	10 at some point during the day	Stand with your feet comfortably apart. Keep your knees soft. Without turning your feet or your knees, rotate from the hips to your left and back to center, then to your right. Remember, these are very small movements; you should rotate your hips a few inches at the most. This is also a wonderful exercise for whenever you are holding your baby.

EXPRESS WORKOUT

Please try not to replace your regular workout with the express version more than once a week.

Perform 20 of each:

1. Pelvic floor warm-up
2. Hand crunch
3. Boomerang
4. Modified push-ups
5. Couch squat
6. At some point later in the day, try 1 set of the cardio block.

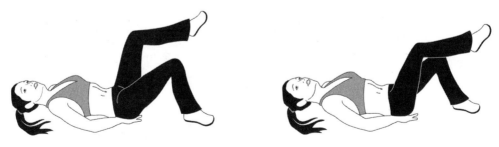

Pelvic tilt with march

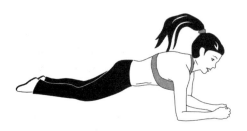

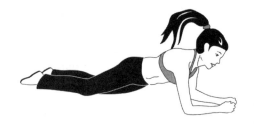

Modified boomerang

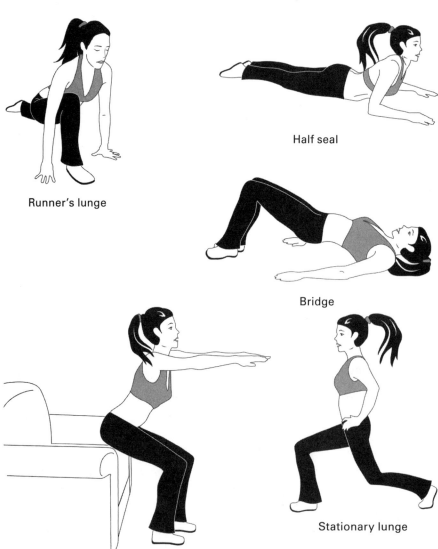

Runner's lunge

Half seal

Bridge

Couch squat

Stationary lunge

Postpartum Depression

Your body needs not only physical healing, but emotional healing!

There is a decreased incidence in postpartum depression when a woman exercises, but only if the exercise is stress relieving and does not cause stress.[40]

After thirty years in the field, my nurse practitioner Susie had seen, heard, and studied it all. And here's what she told me:

In the old days women used to keep babies inside for several months due to fear of the baby catching a virus, which also meant *no* visitors. (Can you imagine how much less stress you would experience without the stress of visitors?) And back in the seventies, women stayed in the hospital for seven days (although I hated the hospital, so that would have pushed me over the edge). PPD has been around for ages, but we see and hear about it more because of all the stress moms put on themselves. (Ever heard of keeping up with the Joneses?)

Postpartum depression is taken very seriously; it affects 20 percent of new mothers. And it affects a higher rate of mothers who underwent in vitro fertilization, like I did. A friend of mine, whom I met through IVF, had a horrible case of it. She couldn't feed her daughter, had no interest at all in her, and contemplated committing suicide on numerous occasions.

Whether you are having minor signs of PPD or severe signs like my friend, or questioning whether you might have it, seek medical attention immediately. You can also find hotlines and anonymous chat groups at apa.org, and nimh.nih.gov.

What causes it? Part of it is hormonal. Your HCG plummets from millions to zero once you push that baby out. How are you supposed to deal with that? If only you had a window to your stomach and could see all the changes your body is going through. Of course, stress is also a factor in PPD. If stress plays a role in your life, take my advice; we'll call it "Lindsay's orders." I was writing this chapter one week after having my first baby and was subject to stress and anxiety like I'd never experienced before—and never want to experience again! Don't do as I did; do as I say. Take the time you need to get mentally and emotionally healthy. There's a good reason why the Family and Medical Leave Act is around—the government understands that women and their mates need time to adjust to having a baby around.

Other factors that may contribute to postpartum depression include:

- Feeling tired after delivery, broken sleep patterns, and not enough rest—these often keep a new mother from regaining her full strength for weeks.
- Low thyroid levels—this can cause symptoms of depression, including depressed mood, decreased interest in things, irritability, fatigue, difficulty concentrating, sleep problems, and weight gain. A simple blood test can determine if this condition is causing a woman's depression. If so, thyroid medicine can be prescribed by a doctor. If you are breastfeeding, you need to run it by your doctor.
- Feeling overwhelmed with a new or another baby to take care of and doubting your ability to be a good mother.
- Feeling stress from changes in work and home routines. Sometimes, women think they have to be Supermom or perfect, which is not realistic and can add stress.
- Feelings of loss—loss of who you are, or were, before having the baby; loss of control; loss of your pre-pregnancy figure; and feeling less attractive.
- Having less free time and less control over time; having to stay home indoors for longer periods of time and having less time to spend with your partner and loved ones.

WHAT ARE SYMPTOMS OF DEPRESSION?

Any of these symptoms during and after pregnancy that last longer than two weeks are signs of depression:

- Restlessness or irritability
- Feeling sad, hopeless, and overwhelmed

- Crying a lot
- Having no energy or motivation
- Eating too little or too much
- Sleeping too little or too much
- Trouble focusing, remembering, or making decisions
- Feeling worthless and guilty
- Loss of interest or pleasure in activities
- Withdrawal from friends and family
- Headaches, chest pain, heart palpitations (the heart beating fast and feeling like it is skipping beats), or hyperventilation (fast and shallow breathing)

After pregnancy, signs of depression may also include being afraid of hurting the baby or oneself and not having any interest in the baby.

THE EDINBURGH POSTNATAL DEPRESSION SCALE

This questionnaire was taken from the *British Journal of Psychiatry* and was developed by J. L. Cox, J. M. Holden, and R. Sagovsky, and is used with their permission.

1. Underline the response which comes closest to how you have been feeling in the previous 7 days.
2. All ten items must be completed.
3. Care should be taken to avoid the possibility of the mother discussing her answers with others.
4. You should complete the scale yourself, unless you have limited English or have difficulty with reading.

As you have recently had a baby, we would like to know how you are feeling. Please UNDERLINE the answer which comes closest to how you have felt IN THE PAST 7 DAYS, not just how you feel today.

1. **I have been able to laugh and see the funny side of things.**
   a. As much as I always could
   b. Not quite so much now
   c. Definitely not so much now
   d. Not at all

2. I have looked forward with enjoyment to things.

   a. As much as I ever did

   b. Rather less than I used to

   c. Definitely less than I used to

   d. Hardly at all

3. I have blamed myself unnecessarily when things went wrong.

   a. Yes, most of the time

   b. Yes, some of the time

   c. Not very often

   d. No, never

4. I have been anxious or worried for no good reason.

   a. No, not at all

   b. Hardly ever

   c. Yes, sometimes

   d. Yes, very often

5. I have felt scared or panicky for no very good reason.

   a. Yes, quite a lot

   b. Yes, sometimes

   c. No, not much

   d. No, not at all

6. Things have been getting on top of me.

   a. Yes, most of the time I haven't been able to cope at all

   b. Yes, sometimes I haven't been coping as well as usual

   c. No, most of the time I have coped quite well

   d. No, I have been coping as well as ever

7. I have been so unhappy that I have had difficulty sleeping.

   a. Yes, most of the time

   b. Yes, sometimes

   c. Not very often

   d. No, not at all

8. I have felt sad or miserable.

   a. Yes, most of the time

   b. Yes, quite often

   c. Not very often

   d. No, not at all

9. I have been so unhappy that I have been crying.

   a. Yes, most of the time

   b. Yes, quite often

c. Only occasionally

d. No, never

10. **The thought of harming myself has occurred to me.**

a. Yes, quite often

b. Sometimes

c. Hardly ever

d. Never

Since I'm not a psychologist, I don't feel comfortable giving you the rating scale, but if you see that you are responding yes to a majority of the questions, it is time for you to contact your doctor and be up-front about what you're experiencing. There is no shame in admitting your feelings—you are not responsible for feeling the way you do, but you are responsible for doing something about it so that you can feel better and enjoy life. If postpartum depression does not affect you, try this test to see if you are a positive or a negative person:

DO YOU HAVE A POSITIVE OR NEGATIVE SELF-IMAGE?

We all do it—we beat up ourselves and our self-image. Take a notepad with you everywhere you go for one day. Write down every thought that pops into your head about yourself and your body. As a mom, you might think that you don't think about yourself throughout the day, but you might be surprised! And if you only have three notes . . . you need to think more about yourself!

Now tally your negative and positive thoughts about yourself. Do your negative thoughts outnumber your positive ones? When it comes to your self-image, are you a negative thinker or positive thinker? If you're a negative thinker, it's time to turn it around. You can improve your self-image by simply thinking better thoughts about yourself. And if you have people in your life who tell you negative things, tell them to shove it!

Phase 3: Condition (and Get Rid of the Jiggly Cellulite!) (Weeks 9–11)

As you make the transition at weeks nine to eleven, you will now be working out four times a week, with an express workout option. If you had a complicated C-section or gave birth to twins, begin this phase during weeks eleven to thirteen. This is the stage when my fertility meds excuse got me in trouble. Remember how my fertility meds made me gain weight? I was back to my pre-pregnancy weight at this point, but I still had ten pounds to go because I hadn't lost my fertility weight. Well, I was the one putting the food in my mouth and not turning off the breast-feeding eating radar! No more excuses. At the end of this stage you should start seeing rapid improvements, including less jiggle, and you'll be closer to that pre-pregnancy weight if you stayed within your recommended weight gain.

If you had a C-section, your swelling should be significantly improved by twelve weeks. Contact your doctor if you are still having pain. Be aware that swelling of the uterus and incision site is not completely reduced by now. Give it six months.

If you gave birth years ago and are using this program, spend two weeks in this phase and add one or two extra days of walking. If you happen to jump into this book and are around six to eight weeks post-pregnancy, *please* make sure you start with Phase 1. Your core muscles need to fire in sequence and get healthy from the inside out first!

"REDUCE YOUR BACK PAIN DURING FEEDINGS"

You can work on relieving your back pain while feeding your baby. One of the keys to this is to switch sides every feeding. Also do the posture check core activation (from weeks zero to four). Just making the tummy muscle work will immediately take strain off your back. Help relieve back pain by also doing spinal flexion and spinal extension in a chair (see page 152).

CFS Phase 3 (Weeks 9–11)

Remember, your body is still recovering. To determine you are doing the correct amount of reps for your body, you should be able to finish one more rep with good form; if not, it's time to back off the number of reps.

Exercise	Sets x Reps/Frequency	How To
Runner's lunge	Hold 20 seconds each leg. M W F	Same as Phase 2.
Pelvic floor warm-up	1 x 10 M W F	Same as Phase 2.
Core activation	1 x 10 M W F	Same as Phase 2.
Hip slings	1 x 20 M W F	Same as Phase 2.
Hand crunch	Beginners: 1 x 30 Veterans: 1 x 40 M W F	Same as Phase 2.
Leg scoot	1 x 10 each side M W F	Start from your pelvic warm-up position, hands to your sides, knees bent. Extend one leg forward by scooting your heel slowly; do not let your back arch. Keep your PF and TA engaged.
Boomerang	1 x 30 M W F	Same as Phase 2, but you can do it from a plank position instead of modifying with your knees down.
Seal	1 x 15 M W F	Same as Phase 2, only now you will lift your lower body off the floor as your upper body shifts toward the floor in a rocking motion.
Modified side plank lifts	1 x 15 M W F	Start in a modified side plank by placing your right hip and knees on the floor. Place your right elbow on the floor and your left hand on the floor in front of you. Lift and lower your left hip.

Exercise	Sets x Reps/Frequency	How To
Two-elbow taps and release	1 x 15 M W F	Sit on your buttocks. Lean back with your elbows at shoulder level and reach. Sit tall and release. See figures on page 232.
Modified push-ups	Beginners: 2 x 10 Veterans: 2 x 20 M W F	Same as Phase 2.
Lunge-plié-lunge	Beginners: 1 x 20 Veterans: 2 x 20 M W F	Begin with a stationary lunge, as you did in Phase 2. Rotate to the center so you're facing forward, and perform a plié squat. Rotate your body and perform a stationary lunge in the other direction. See figures on page 232.
Modified dips	Beginners: 1 x 10 Veterans: 2 x 10 M W F	Sit on a sturdy chair with your hands flat beside your hips. Using your arms, lift your hips off the chair and walk your feet forward two feet. Bend your elbows to ninety degrees and extend. If your wrists bother you, place weights underneath your hands and grip them as you perform the dips. See figures on page 232.
Squat to overhead press	2 x 15 M W F	Same as you did in the second trimester, page 132. Beginners and veterans, use 3- to 8-pound weights.
Cardio block	M W F Try to finish 20 reps within 1 minute. Beginners: 1–2 sets Veterans: 2–3 sets	Same as Phase 2.

Exercise	Sets x Reps/Frequency	How To
Cardio only: If you're unable to go outside or use a treadmill, do 2–3 sets of the cardio block.	T Th	30-minute walk. Beginners: Add 1 minute of jogging every 6 minutes. Veterans: Add 1 minute of jogging every 3 minutes.
Hot potato	During the day	Every time you hold your baby, do the core activation exercise and pull your abs away from the baby.
Kegels	3 x 10 at bedtime	See page 82 for description.

EXPRESS WORKOUT

Please try not to replace your regular workout with the express version more than once a week.

Perform 20 of each:

1. Pelvic floor warm-up
2. Hand crunch
3. Modified side plank lifts
4. Modified push-up
5. Squat and press
6. At a point later in the day, try to do 1 set of the cardio block.

Why do we do intervals when we do cardio? Plain and simple: You burn more calories—sometimes twice as many—doing an interval cardio workout. Who doesn't want to spend thirty minutes instead of an hour burning three hundred calories?

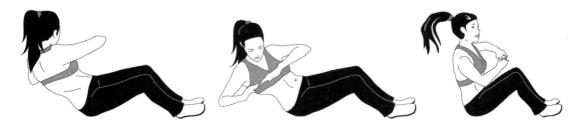

Two-elbow taps and release

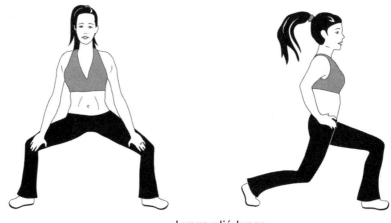

Lunge-plié-lunge

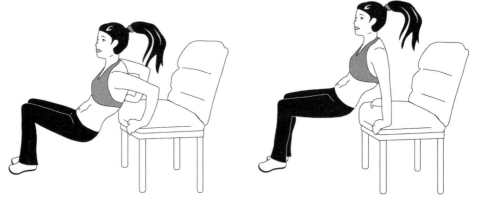

Modified dips

Still having back pain? Make sure you have ruled out diastasis recti (consult page 84). If you do not have diastasis, make sure to go back to Phase 1 or 2 and master the moves before moving on.

FIND THE TIME

Now, how do you find time to squeeze exercise in? Put the baby in a carrier and take a walk or do some lunges and squats. Call a neighbor—relieve your stress by getting out of the house. Do you have three kids at home—one grabbing your leg, the other yelling "Mom!" and the baby crying for food? Put the two older ones in a stroller (as long as they're not too big), strap the baby in a carrier, and get some fresh air!

At about three or four months post-pregnancy, returning to your pre-pregnancy weight is a good milestone. Now do you have your pre-pregnancy figure? We'll get there with the next stage! Even if your weight is the same as pre-pregnancy, that belly may still need a little work. Don't worry, it's the number one complaint with moms, and you're taking the right steps to get your figure back too!

Phase 4: Shrink (Weeks 12–14)

If you had a vaginal birth, then it is recommended that you enter this phase during weeks twelve to fourteen post-pregnancy. For C-sections and twin gestations (vaginal or C-section), you should enter this between weeks fourteen and sixteen.

Exercise	Sets x Reps/Frequency	How To
Runner's lunge	Hold 20 seconds each leg. M W F	Same as Phase 3.
Pelvic floor warm-up	1 x 10 M W F	Same as Phase 3.
Core activation	1 x 10 M W F	Same as Phase 3.
Hip slings	1 x 20 M W F	Same as Phase 3.
Opposite arm and leg reach	1 x 15 each side M W F	Start on your back with your knees bent. Extend your right arm straight over your head while simultaneously extending your left leg at a forty-five-degree angle. Switch sides. See figure on page 237.
Flight	2 x 30 seconds M W F	Lie on your stomach with your arms to your sides and your thumbs pointed up. Lock your legs and lift your upper and lower body off the floor. See figure on page 237.
Butterfly crunch	Beginners: 30 Veterans: 2 x 30 M W F	Start in the crunch position with the soles of your feet together in a butterfly position. Perform a Kegel and then a pelvic tilt as you crunch up, being careful not to pooch your belly out. Release the pelvic tilt and Kegel, and then release the crunch. See figure on page 237.

Exercise	Sets x Reps/Frequency	How To
Asymmetrical push-up	Beginners: 2 x 10 Veterans: 2 x 20 M W F	Stagger your hands so one hand is in front of the other in a modified plank position (knees down). Perform 10 push-ups before switching your hand position so the other hand is placed above shoulder level. Veterans' modification: Lift your knees off the floor. See figures on page 237.
Mermaid	Beginners: 1 x 15 Veterans: 1 x 20 M W F	Start in a side plank. Lift and lower your hips. If this is too difficult, hold a side plank. See figures on page 238.
Plank clock	Start with 5 reps on each side and work up to 10. M W F	Start in a plank position, which you can modify by placing your knees on the floor as in the modified boomerang in Phase 2. Imagine a clock on the floor; your shoulders are the center. Move your right hand to 12 o'clock, 3 o'clock, and 6 o'clock. Repeat with your left hand. See figures on page 238.
Lunge core twist	1 x 20 M W F	From a standing position with feet together, clasp your hands with straight arms at shoulder height to your left. Step forward and lunge with your right leg, rotate from the waist, and twist to the right. Veterans: Use 3- to 8-pound weights. See figures on page 238.
Squat and press	2 x 20 M W F	Same as Phase 3.

Exercise	Sets x Reps/Frequency	How To
Dips	Beginners: 1 x 10 Veterans: 2 x 10 M W F	Similar to modified dips on page 232, but this is the advanced version. Sit on a sturdy chair with your hands flat beside your hips. Using your arms, lift your hips off the chair and walk your feet forward until your legs are straight. If your wrists bother you, place weights underneath your hands and grip them as you perform the dips. See figure on page 239.
Core biceps	2 x 15 M W F	From a standing position, lift and hold one knee up as you perform biceps curls. Switch legs for each set. Beginners and veterans, use 3- to 8-pound weights.
Cardio Block	M W F Try to finish 20 reps within 1 minute. Beginners: 2 sets Veterans: 3 sets	Same as Phase 2.
Cardio Only: If you're unable to go outside or use a treadmill, do 2–3 sets of the cardio block.	T Th	30-minute walk. Beginners: Add 1 minute of jogging every 4 minutes. Veterans: Alternate 1 minute of jogging with 1 minute of walking.
Kegels	3 x 10 at bedtime	See page 82.

EXPRESS WORKOUT

Please try not to replace your regular workout with the express version more than once a week.

Perform 20 of each:

1. Pelvic floor warm-up
2. Butterfly crunch
3. Asymmetrical push-up
4. Plank clock
5. Squat and press
6. At a point later in the day, try to do 1 set of the cardio block.

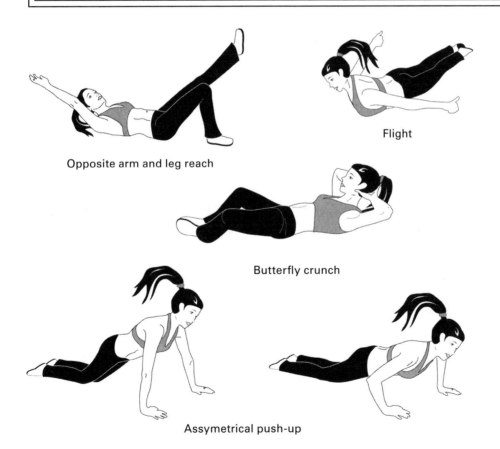

Opposite arm and leg reach

Flight

Butterfly crunch

Assymetrical push-up

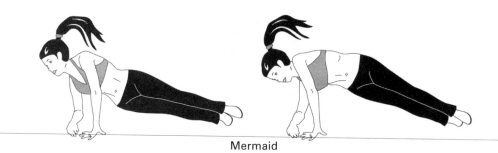

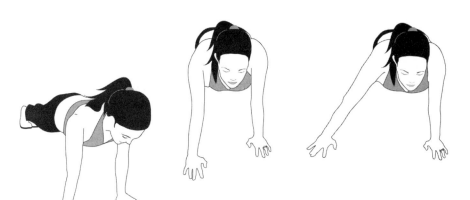

Mermaid

Plank clock

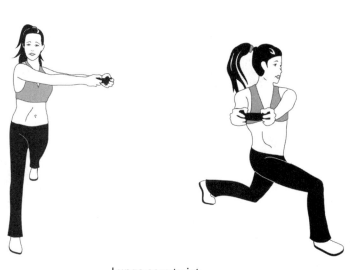

Lunge core twist

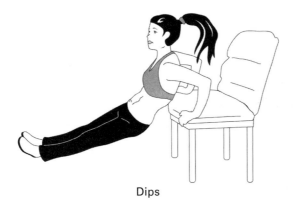

Dips

Remember, you have to do cardio to get rid of the overlying fat and see your abs.

Your baby will start to be a little less clingy and have a sleep schedule nailed down. . . . Well, almost.

Stop strolling and start moving! Squeeze the buncakes as you walk. Imagine a pencil has been put under them and every time you take a step you must squeeze that pencil! This is good for—guess what? The buncakes! And it will get your heart racing, which in turn burns calories.

At this point you are more than likely starting to feel "normal." And most likely you will need more of a workout by now for the total body, especially if you've been consistent. Bump up the calorie burn and toning by going to Part III, or if you're ready you can use my *Boot Camp 2* DVD, with ten-minute workouts including cardio and toning! Use coupon code "bookdvd20" for 20 percent off.

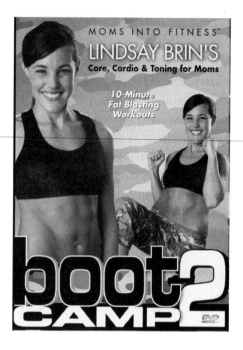

MOMS INTO FITNESS™
LINDSAY BRIN'S
Core, Cardio & Toning for Moms

10-Minute
Fat Blasting
Workouts

boot CAMP 2
DVD

Remember that it is easier to make the time than it is to find excuses! I've given you all kinds of suggestions to modify the program to fit your schedule. Now it's up to you to make the commitment. That said: You will be tired! Among all these new (or old, if you have more than one child) experiences, you are throwing another wrench into the works. After the initial high of working out, you will be tired. But your body will get used to *all* of the demands soon. And if not, you need to slow down. This is when you may have to recruit your husband, partner, neighbor, or a grandparent to take care of the baby during or after your workout, especially during the first three months of your baby's life—they love and have to be cuddled constantly!

NO TIME TO EXERCISE?

Here are four exercises you can do with your baby. I ask that you only sub these exercises up to once a week, or not at all if possible. You will see more results from following the program, but I know we all need some slack in our hectic schedules!

Four exercises you can do with your baby:

1. Squat and press: works the shoulders, core, lower body
2. Pelvic rotations (as discussed in CFS method): works the core
3. Teasers: works the core, arms
4. Reverse crunches: works the core. Lie on your back and bring your knees toward your chest. Hold baby on his or her stomach on your shins, and move your legs back and forth slightly.

The first three are found at youtube.com/momsintofitness.
Your baby must have good head control and some core strength to participate in these exercises.

PART III

Lifestyle

· 10 ·

STARVED FOR SLEEP, BUT TIME FOR EXERCISE

I sometimes wear my pj's all day and love being a homebody. I love watching movies on the weekend with my hubby (and sometimes in our room by myself) and not leaving the house on Sundays, except for church. But fitness is a part of my everyday—well, almost everyday—regimen. Whether it's taking the stroller around the neighborhood, joining my HIIT (high-intensity interval training) group at five a.m. Wednesdays, or kicking my own butt by doing my *Postnatal Boot Camp* DVD, I get it done. Why? Exercise makes me feel better, and when I feel better, everyone in my house does. There have been a number of times when my husband has dangled my workout shoes in front of me, which means, "You are cranky—please go work out so when you come back you are pleasant to be around." I don't need the reminder often, but it's good to have a supportive team on your side—especially on those cranky-pants days.

If you are reading this after recently having a baby, then you know what I mean. The good thing is your newborn is now on more of a schedule. Four months made a huge difference for me—in my body and in my baby. It was a time I felt like I was in control again, or somewhat in control. The parade of friends and family had been reduced from a marching band to a lone clown on a unicycle—and, speaking of cycles, you may begin menstruating again if you've stopped breast-feeding, and your body is beginning to resemble, in operation if not in appearance, what it was pre-pregnancy. Now is the time to make the switch, mentally and physically, from nutrition and exercise being a transitional phase to being a permanent part of your lifestyle.

The good news about making fitness a part of your lifestyle? The more active you are, the less fat you store. And when it comes to nutrition, if you can concentrate on the food you are eating instead of shoving food in when you have a few free minutes, you will more easily lose weight and keep it off. The key in the lifestyle phase is to get into a regular routine.

THE TOP SIX EXCUSES NOT TO WORK OUT

1. **My baby didn't sleep well and I only got three hours of sleep.** This is the one time I will tell you to not work out!
2. **I work full-time in addition to being a mom.** Try ten to twenty minutes before work—you'll start your day off on the right foot!
3. **I don't have the energy.** Remember, exercise energizes you!
4. **I don't have time.** Tell your partner he or she's in charge for twenty minutes when he or she gets home.
5. **Working out is *boring*.** So not everybody enjoys working out—in fact, probably only 20 percent of people enjoy it. But 100 percent of people love the benefits of working out! You do the laundry even though it's boring . . . because you have to!
6. **The top excuse: Being pregnant made me gain too much weight.** Unless you were on bed rest, this is not an excuse. If you gained eighty pounds during pregnancy, that wasn't the baby's fault!

It takes three weeks for something to become a habit, and it takes three weeks to break a habit. I don't know how scientifically verifiable that is, but based on my experience it makes sense. Getting into a new routine is hard, but if you can get past that twenty-one-day mark, it seems to be much easier to maintain (which is also the reason we switch our workouts every two to three weeks). So, for now, your first goal is to commit to sticking with my program for twenty-one days. Here's a simple process for achieving just about anything in life:

1. Set goals.
2. Write them down.
3. Develop a plan.
4. Execute that plan.
5. Reevaluate that timeline so it all can get done.

Goal Sheet

How soon should you plan to return to your pre-pregnancy weight?

1. Pre-pregnancy weight____ (And be truthful—how much did you weigh the day you found out you were pregnant, not the months leading up to it?)
2. Weight gained during pregnancy____
3. Timeline____
   If you gained your recommended amount of weight, your goal is five months.
   If you gained ten to fifteen pounds on top of your recommended amount, your goal is six to nine months.
   If you gained sixteen to thirty pounds on top of your recommended amount, your goal is nine to twelve months.
4. What is your fitness goal? Getting to the top of the stairs without being winded? Or finishing this workout without taking a number of breaks?
5. Define success for yourself, not by anyone else's standards.
   Is success to you being a full-time mom?
   Is success to you having a part-time job in addition to being a mom?
   Is success to you moving up in the workforce in addition to being mom?
   You have to fulfill your dreams. And hopefully your partner or another family member can help support that.

Your body is a fat-burning machine within six months of having a baby. Take advantage of it! It is possible to have a better body than ever, but you must be conscious of losing too much weight.

6. Short-term goal:
7. Long-term goal:
   You *will* stall out on the scale. Put it away, keep exercising, and it will change next week; I promise.
   Take measurements and weight every week for small victories and goals. You will find your Progress Tracker on the following page.
8. Target weight____ (please use the calculation on page 249 or simply go to momsintofitness.com/weight-loss-calculator and plug in a few numbers)

In addition to your Goal Sheet, I also want you to use this Progress Tracker I'm sure you might decide this should go in Part 2, but when did you want to start really tracking your results? Or have the time to do so?

Measure yourself every Monday morning at the same time. You will be measuring the largest circumference of that area unless otherwise noted.

Weight__
Neck__
Shoulders__
Chest/back__
Natural waistline__ (this is the smallest part of your waist)
1" below navel__
Hips__
Thigh__
Calf__

Make a Plan

Here is an ideal week:

Monday: Stroller 10 Interval workout
Tuesday: Cardio interval
Wednesday: Stroller 10 Interval workout
Thursday: Cardio interval or rest
Friday: Interval workout (this can come from one of my *Boot Camp* DVDs or using the Stroller 10)
Saturday: Family exercise
Sunday: Rest; plan and cook meals for the week

Each of your Monday through Friday workouts will last from thirty to fifty-five minutes.

There is an express workout available, just like in the other parts of the book!

Your Saturday family exercise is up to you in terms of content and length. I'll provide much more detail about these workouts in the pages that follow.

Refining Your Goal and Your Body

In addition to committing to the workout schedule above, you need to set a more long-term goal. I've already asked you to choose an outfit you'd like to be able to fit into, but now it's time to get a bit more specific and scientific about your goals. For years, we've concentrated on reaching a target weight. Want to weigh X pounds by Y date is not a bad way to put a carrot out in front of yourself. There is a better way, and the good news is that it is also a fairer way of determining what is healthy and right for your body type.

Body mass index (BMI) is a measurement that accounts for both your height and weight and how they work together proportionally. I'm sure you've heard someone described as "big boned"—well, that is true. Some of us have smaller frames than others, so even though two people can be the same height, that doesn't mean a weight that is healthy, desirable, and achievable for one is right for the other. BMI provides you with a range of weights that account for those differences in the amounts of fat and muscle we each carry on our bodies.

The body mass index chart on page 248 will help you find your body mass index. Find your height in the top rows—expressed either in inches or in feet and inches. Once you've found your height, find where your weight and height intersect. The number in the box is your BMI.

We're going to use your BMI as a way to gauge your progress—to determine where you are today and to set a goal for where you want to be down the line. Because you were recently pregnant or you haven't worked out since you were pregnant, your BMI is probably going to be higher than what you'd like. That's OK. The goal here is to improve and use that as a motivation to get your BMI back into the healthy range.

Finding Your Goal BMI

OK, so you know what your BMI is, but what does that do for you? Well, as the following chart shows, your BMI places you in a particular category. For

BMI	Height (in)																		
	58	59	60	61	62	63	64	65	66	67	68	69	70	71	72	73	74	75	76
Wgt. (lbs)	4'10"	4'11"	5'0"	5'1"	5'2"	5'3"	5'4"	5'5"	5'6"	5'7"	5'8"	5'9"	5'10"	5'11"	6'0"	6'1"	6'2"	6'3"	6'4"
100	21	20	20	19	18	18	17	17	16	16	15	15	14	14	14	13	13	13	12
105	22	21	21	20	19	19	18	18	17	16	16	16	15	15	14	14	14	13	13
110	23	22	22	21	20	20	19	18	18	17	17	16	16	15	15	15	14	14	13
115	24	23	23	22	21	20	20	19	19	18	18	17	17	16	16	15	15	14	14
120	25	24	23	23	22	21	21	20	19	19	18	18	17	17	16	16	15	15	15
125	26	25	24	24	23	22	22	21	20	20	19	18	18	17	17	17	16	16	15
130	27	26	25	25	24	23	22	22	21	20	20	19	19	18	18	17	17	16	16
135	28	27	26	26	25	24	23	23	22	21	21	20	19	19	18	18	17	17	16
140	29	28	27	27	26	25	24	23	23	22	21	21	20	20	19	19	18	18	17
145	30	29	28	27	27	26	25	24	23	23	22	21	21	20	20	19	19	18	18
150	31	30	29	28	27	27	26	25	24	24	23	22	22	21	20	20	19	19	18
155	32	31	30	29	28	28	27	26	25	24	24	23	22	22	21	20	20	19	19
160	34	32	31	30	29	28	28	27	26	25	24	24	23	22	22	21	21	20	20
165	35	33	32	31	30	29	28	28	27	26	25	24	24	23	22	22	21	21	20
170	36	34	33	32	31	30	29	28	27	27	26	25	24	24	23	22	22	21	21
175	37	35	34	33	32	31	30	29	28	27	27	26	25	24	24	23	23	22	21
180	38	36	35	34	33	32	31	30	29	28	27	27	26	25	24	24	23	23	22
185	39	37	36	35	34	33	32	31	30	29	28	27	27	26	25	24	24	23	23
190	40	38	37	36	35	34	33	32	31	30	29	28	27	27	26	25	24	24	23
195	41	39	38	37	36	35	34	33	32	31	30	29	28	27	27	26	25	24	24
200	42	40	39	38	37	36	34	33	32	31	30	30	29	28	27	26	26	25	24
205	43	41	40	39	38	36	35	34	33	32	31	30	29	29	28	27	26	26	25
210	44	43	41	40	38	37	36	35	34	33	32	31	30	29	29	28	27	26	26
215	45	44	42	41	39	38	37	36	35	34	33	32	31	30	29	28	28	27	26
220	46	45	43	42	40	39	38	37	36	35	34	33	32	31	30	29	28	28	27
225	47	46	44	43	41	40	39	38	36	35	34	33	32	31	31	30	29	28	27
230	48	47	45	44	42	41	40	38	37	36	35	34	33	32	31	30	30	29	28
235	49	48	46	44	43	42	40	39	38	37	36	35	34	33	32	31	30	29	29
240	50	49	47	45	44	43	41	40	39	38	37	36	35	34	33	32	31	30	29
245	51	50	48	46	45	43	42	41	40	38	37	36	35	34	33	32	32	31	30
250	52	51	49	47	46	44	43	42	40	39	38	37	36	35	34	33	32	31	30
255	53	52	50	48	47	45	44	43	41	40	39	38	37	36	35	34	33	32	31
260	54	53	51	49	48	46	45	43	42	41	40	38	37	36	35	34	33	33	32
265	56	54	52	50	49	47	46	44	43	42	40	39	38	37	36	35	34	33	32
270	57	55	53	51	49	48	46	45	44	42	41	40	39	38	37	36	35	34	33
275	58	56	54	52	50	49													

each height and weight combination, your number corresponds to a particular designation. Obviously, you want your BMI to fall into the Normal range:

BMI	Category
18.5 or less	Underweight
18.6 to 24.9	Normal
25.0 to 29.9	Overweight
30.0 to 39.9	Obese
40 or greater	Very Obese

Record your target BMI here: _____

Getting to Your Target BMI

If your BMI is not in the Normal range, the next step is to find your target weight. To set your target BMI, choose a BMI in the Normal category closest to your current BMI. Once you have determined your healthy BMI, use the following formula to find your target weight.

(target BMI) x (height in inches x height in inches) / 703 = target weight

As you can see, weight isn't unimportant, but you have to put it into some kind of context. Add your target BMI and your target weight to your Goal Sheet. Later on you can refine your target weight, but for now your goal is to get into the Normal BMI range. If you already are and you want to lose additional pounds, then set a target weight goal that is the lowest that will keep you in the Normal range and won't cause you to slip into the Underweight category. You can also calculate your target weight at www.momsintofitness.com/weight-loss-calculator.

MORE ON BODY FAT AND METABOLISM

If you've got a little extra time in your busy schedule and are interested in learning more about your metabolism and how your body sheds weight, check out my book *The Cheerleader Fitness Plan*. As a veteran NFL cheerleader, I figured I would give you the tricks of the trade. Just how do NFL cheerleaders fit into tiny two-pieces every Sunday afternoon?

You don't have to be a cheerleader to read *The Cheerleader Fitness Plan*. It will give you an interval workout for six weeks, and every week we switch it up so your body doesn't get bored. And it provides a little insight into the lives of real NFL cheerleaders, and how the NFL moms do it all—plus lots of secrets on losing weight for the coveted calendar shoot!

Instead of getting into too much science, since I know your time is limited, we're just going to dive right into some quick tips on what works. And it's what works for moms! I know you can't—or don't want to—make a four-course meal of tofu, broccoli, salad, and green tea. So I will teach you tricks you can quickly read through and instantly put into your everyday life.

LOSE WEIGHT WITHOUT EXERCISING!

Of course, if you exercise you will lose it a lot faster.

Here are twelve weight-loss rules every mom should know. And you should start today!

1. Eat high-volume foods such as soups, salads, vegetables, and lean protein. You will be satisfied with fewer calories!

2. Use the "plate method": Make your main dish vegetables instead of meat. Fill half your plate with vegetables, which you will eat first, then a quarter of your plate with lean protein and a quarter of your plate with whatever you wish. And add an eight-ounce glass of skim milk if you need some extra calcium. If you do this for a few days, you'll lose immediately!

3. Get rid of empty calories. A calorie is a calorie, but I call it empty because it has no nutrients or vitamins and doesn't fill you up. Do not drink your calories—eliminate the regular soda and alcohol if you've still got a lot of weight to lose. But if you can't live without it, make sure your beverage of choice is less than 150 calories a day.

4. Sit while eating, and eat slowly. This eliminates the mindless eating that happens when you pass by the pantry or the candy jar at work. Oh, and when you are getting crackers out for your kids, you don't need to grab a few for yourself, unless it is your snack time. Even if the baby starts crying during dinner, *do not* scarf your food down!

5. No eating after dinner. Get into a fat-burning zone while sleeping and burn through stored fat, not fat you just ate. It does not matter when you eat the calories—a calorie is a calorie, no matter what time of day—but after dinner is when most moms give into temptation and eat a majority of them.

HOW TO AVOID EATING AT NIGHT

- Go to bed early.
- Spend the rest of the evening in your bedroom, where food is off-limits.
- Take a relaxing bath.
- Drink some hot tea for a little or zero-calorie beverage.

6. No BLTs. That means *no* bites, licks, or tastes. Savor one snack you really like. And no eating the leftovers off your child's plate—not even a bite! For less temptation, buy just one snack food at the store each week.

7. When eating out, take half of your plate home. Have it boxed up before you even get your meal.

8. Drink one glass of water before every meal or snack. It will help you feel full and flush fat. Hate water? Try Vitaminwater or a lemonade mixture with less than ten calories per serving.

9. Use the five-minute trick: Wait five minutes before giving in to temptation—do some deep breathing, go to another room, go on a walk, or if you're at home with the kids, do a few minutes of squats or run up and down the stairs (you may not even want that tempting treat after that!).

10. Unfortunately, you cannot give in to every temptation and lose weight. But you should give in to your cravings once a week.

11. Get your z's. Studies show getting enough sleep can help curb your hunger. I was watching *Oprah* one day and it really caught my attention when Dr. Oz said there is such a thing as a "mommy brain." During pregnancy your brain shrinks by 8 percent, but then quickly reestablishes itself for all the new tasks you will be doing with a new baby. So if you become a little forgetful, blame it on the mommy brain! But the brain does not grow without sleep, so it's important to get your z's. Dr. Oz also said to take your omega-3 fatty acids, because the baby steals yours—this helps your brain as well.

12. *And the biggest rule:* Do not let one mistake sabotage your goal! Make up for your splurge at your next meal by eating all veggies, which is virtually a calorie-free meal.

Would you rather have a handful of candy corns? Or six cups of popped popcorn? And don't say you'd like to have them together. . . .

Six cups of popped popcorn has the same amount of calories as a handful of candy corn. More specifically, fifteen pieces of candy corn equals six cups of air-popped popcorn or four cups of healthy buttered microwave popcorn (about 150 calories). The popcorn will fill you up with fewer calories.

> Is a doughnut staring you right in the face?
>
> So it's not mealtime and you've already had your one snack for the day. But there is a doughnut sitting on the office counter or kitchen table and it's staring you right in the face. What do you do? Well, if you are a mom who is not busy (I have yet to meet an "un-busy" mom) and you have an extra hour to do cardio, go for it. But if you're a busy mom, get it out of your sight!

> Overeating has a lot to do with your environment. So clean up your environment! Get rid of candy jars, cookies, or a pantry full of sugary snacks. Drive a different route that doesn't take you past the fast-food places. If there's a vending machine in the office kitchen that gets you every time, or if the cafeteria offers a lot of fattening foods, stay away from those places.

Pregorexia

Pregorexia is similar to anorexia but occurs during and after pregnancy. Approximately 5 percent of women from every walk of life will suffer from this unnatural desire not to gain the twenty-five to thirty-five pounds that doctors recommend. Like postpartum depression, pregorexia can be brought on by the stresses associated with carrying and giving birth to a child. There's no shame in admitting that you are struggling with this issue. As much as I focus on not gaining too much weight during pregnancy and shedding those pounds afterward, I don't want you to believe that you are under such pressure that you wind up gaining too little weight or not eating enough postpregnancy. A new mother should *never* consume fewer than eight hundred calories. Consistently falling below that number and not gaining sufficient weight during pregnancy can lead to a low-birth-weight baby. Babies born with a low birth weight are prone to the following physical and developmental problems:

- anemia
- ADHD
- rickets
- heart disease
- depression
- poor growth and cognitive development

If you find yourself in the position of not eating enough or purging, consult with your physician immediately.

> Eat right every chance you get! If you're eating while standing up, driving the car, or on the go, you'll never feel like you've eaten. Sit down while eating—you'll be less apt to snack on a bunch of junk between meals.

"Normal" Calorie Consumption

OK, we've looked at your body composition and set goals for your BMI and weight. How many calories should you be consuming in order achieve those goals? Remember when we were calculating basal metabolic rate, body mass index, and the like? Now is when you need to do these calculations for yourself to get an even better idea of the difference between what you should be consuming and what you are consuming.

> ### Reading Labels to Determine Calorie Count
>
> Reading labels can be confusing sometimes. So break it down and just look at calories, sodium, sugar, and fiber. I'll bet a fried chimichanga or cheesy lasagna frozen meal will not be low in calories, so be smart. Make sure the calories fit within your calorie budget for *one* serving.

BMR is the minimum number of calories you need for basic life-sustaining activities, such as breathing, drinking, and eating. Here is the formula for determining your BMR:

English BMR Formula

Women: BMR = 655 + (4.35 x weight in pounds) +
(4.7 x height in inches) – (4.7 x age in years)

Men: BMR = 66 + (6.23 x weight in pounds) +
(12.7 x height in inches) – (6.8 x age in years)

Enter your BMR here: _____.

You can plug in your height and weight at www.momsintofitness.com/weight-loss-calculator and have your BMR calculated for you.

An Easier BMR Calculation

Did the section above have your head spinning? I hope not, but if it did, here's a simpler way to estimate your BMR, or how many calories you burn daily without exercise:

How much do you weigh? _____
Add a zero your weight: _____
Add your weight to that number: _____
Total = BMR: _____

For example, if you weigh 160 pounds, you add a zero to come up with 1,600. Next, add your weight to that number to get 1,760 calories burned per day, or your BMR. Keep in mind that this simpler method doesn't accurately account for how active you are. Also, be aware that most of us tend to underestimate the number of calories we consume. And estimates can have a real effect on how successful you are in getting to your ideal weight and shape, so if it's at all possible, do the more strenuous calculations. Monitor your success (and non-success) on page 246 with the Progress Tracker.

As you move through my program, some of those numbers will change as you lose weight. For example, any calculation you did that involves your weight should be adjusted after you do your weekly weigh-in.

Now that you know what your goals are and you have a general idea of what your weekly exercise plan is going to look like, we'll turn to the specifics of your workout and nutrition in the next chapter.

· 11 ·

KICKING IT INTO GEAR

Nutrition in 5-4-3-2-1 and the

Stroller 10

Have you ever wondered if it's your willpower standing between you and the body you've always wanted? Well, the good news is you can increase your willpower, but it's hard work. And let me tell you, many women do not succeed on willpower alone. So let's use motivation, such as your skinny jeans, a swimsuit, or purely wanting more energy to run after the kids! Either way, I don't want to hear "I just don't have the willpower to stick to it." This plan is catered to your lifestyle and every minute you do not have. And let me remind you that excuses don't help you lose weight.

You will be working your core muscles, doing cardiovascular work, and using stretching and yoga moves to lengthen your muscles. The cardio work that you will be doing is based on the premise of getting you the maximum workout in the minimum amount of time through interval training. (Interval training is the most effective means for you to get into your fat-burning zone and increase your cardiovascular efficiency.) The exercises are all easy to do, and many include using your baby's stroller, so you can also maximize the time you spend with your new baby and your other children if you have them.

I'm not going to give you elaborate meal plans. What I will provide is something you can easily incorporate into your life today—without making too many adjustments, preparing new grocery lists, and so on.

My Palm Plan makes eating the right amount and the right foods fast and easy. As a part of my shortcut, you will measure the amount you eat using the palm method. If you open your hand, palm up, and curl your fingers slightly to form a small cup, that is one serving or portion that you should consume. Using this method will give you an approximate "correct" portion of each item from the food groups listed below.

The key is *balance*. In the meals I've provided in this book, I make sure you get your fruits and vegetables, carbs, protein, and even some fat (not too much!).

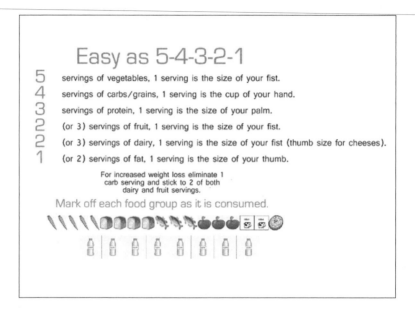

Easy as 5-4-3-2-1

5 servings of vegetables, 1 serving is the size of your fist.
4 servings of carbs/grains, 1 serving is the cup of your hand.
3 servings of protein, 1 serving is the size of your palm.
2 (or 3) servings of fruit, 1 serving is the size of your fist.
2 (or 3) servings of dairy, 1 serving is the size of your fist (thumb size for cheeses).
1 (or 2) servings of fat, 1 serving is the size of your thumb.

For increased weight loss eliminate 1 carb serving and stick to 2 of both dairy and fruit servings.

Mark off each food group as it is consumed.

Five rules that go with this food journal:

1. Drink one glass (one cup or eight ounces) of water before a meal and one glass of water during a meal. You can flavor your water with low-calorie packets such as Crystal Light Lemonade. Tea is also considered water if it's caffeine-free.
2. Eat only during meal and snack times—ideally three meals and one to two snacks or five mini meals, as discussed previously.
3. Of course you can eat out! But be smart and check off some vegetable groups while you're there.
4. Red meat should be consumed no more than one or two times per week. Protein is also found in beans, cheeses, nuts, eggs, chicken, seafood, pork chops, and deli meats.
5. Limit sodium.

The Food Journal

Let's be honest, being a mother and keeping track of a food journal is next to impossible. So all I ask is that you do it for six days. Find out what your weaknesses are and when they occur. If your weakness is after-dinner snacks, look at my ideas on page 264 to eliminate these calories. If chocolate is your weakness, hide it or don't buy it! Also check to see if you're eating the calories to stay in the range of your BMR.

Some Things to Note

My suggested intake above doesn't list any calorie-rich beverages such as regular soda, fruit juice, or alcohol. It also doesn't include potato chips, cookies, and alcoholic beverages or other empty-calorie foods. Just because they aren't specifically mentioned doesn't mean they are forbidden—I just ask you to cut back and to keep track of them in your food journal. Some of us have that salty-oily craving going on, while others have a sweet tooth. In general, you should limit your consumption of simple sugars and/or salty-oilies to less than 150 calories a day. If you can't quit, at least commit to cutting back.

I'm not going to spend much more time than it takes to make this statement: Many of us have a complicated psychological relationship with food and eating. I'm not here to deal with a lot of those issues. I'm incredibly sympathetic and understand that we all bring those issues to the table every time we eat. For the purposes of this chapter, we're going to set those issues aside and deal with the facts about food and its relationship to fitness. We're going to take a more scientific and clinical approach to reduce, as much as we possibly can, all the extra baggage that comes with eating and our emotional attachments to that act.

The Science of Losing a Pound

As I've said, it's all about the calories. So let's talk a bit about what a calorie is. A calorie is a unit of measurement. If you know Spanish, you know the word *calor* means "heat"; the English word *calorie* is derived from the same Latin root. In scientific terms, a calorie is equal to the amount of heat necessary to raise one kilogram of water one degree Celsius.

What it really measures, then, is the amount of energy a food contains. Do you remember how your high school physics teacher defined energy? If he or she was anything like mine, you were probably too distracted by the bad hair and clothes. For that reason, I'll tell you.

Energy = the ability to do work

1 unit of energy = 1 kcal (or calorie)

In other words, calories power all of the physical processes of the body. Basically, they give us energy to function. So when you're scanning nutritional labels on a package, you're getting the measurement of that food's energy content. Generally, that measure is for one hundred grams of a typical serving size of that food. Your body uses the energy contained in the food you eat to fuel the various processes that sustain life and activities beyond mere survival. Any excess calories you take in are stored in the body as fat.

It's not an exact science, but since all the calculations are done the same way across the industry, what matters most is that you understand what a calorie is and what it represents: energy to be used for work.

A Day of Ideal Eating

Remember, I'm all about better and best choices, so this is the best-case scenario for you. You should consume three small meals and one snack, or five mini-meals. If you are a small- to medium-size woman your BMR is likely to fall within a range of eleven hundred to sixteen hundred calories. If you are a large-framed woman, you will need to consume more, so I recommend that you have one additional hand-cup portion of starch and one additional portion of protein. You should never consume fewer than one thousand calories.

If the idea of counting calories and food journaling is daunting, you can use the 60 Day Slimdown Plan on my Web site. But let me warn you, at some point you will have to learn how to count calories for yourself and your family. So just suck it up for a few weeks, learn the ropes, and benefit from it for the rest of your life.

Do you need more energy to get through your day? Whether you are a homemaker, have a full-time job, or are pregnant with your first child, you need energy to get through your day. Your metabolism is what converts stored energy for your daily functions such as walking, eating, exercising, and breathing. By following my exercise plan and using these nutrition ideas, you'll be fueling your body with stuff that will make you feel energized instead of blah.

APPROXIMATE CALORIE CONSUMPTION FROM EACH GROUP

You can skip this next section for time-constraint reasons, but if you ever want to teach your kids good principles and stay off the yo-yo wagon, you need to buck up and learn about calories! I promise it will become a habit after reading labels a few times and measuring your pasta or chicken with the palm method so you can eyeball your servings from here on out.

It is obvious, but I have to repeat this: It's not just how much, but what you eat that will make the difference in effectively, safely, and healthfully losing weight. Here's what you should be consuming from each group:

Vegetables: Those five servings will account for 150 to 200 calories. One half cup of cooked veggies or one cup of raw veggies is approximately 30 calories. That's a lot of food in terms of weight, but not a lot in terms of calories. That's why I recommend you eat more vegetables. They create a lot of bulk in your stomach so you feel fuller, but they don't add a high calorie count.

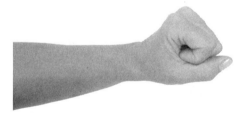

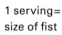
1 serving=
size of fist

Lindsay's Plate Balance Secret

At nearly every meal, half of your plate should be covered with vegetables. That way, you are sure to be getting the proper balance of nutrients, eating the correct number of calories, and consuming enough "bulk" that you will feel full without excessive calories.

Fruits: Your three servings of fruits will have you consuming between 180 and three hundred calories. As you can see, that's comparatively a lot more calories than vegetables. You can eat two more servings of vegetables and still end up a hundred calories or so short of the number of calories you'd consume from eating fruit. Why? Generally, fruits have a higher sugar content than vegetables. Those sugars are good sources of energy and are therefore more calorie rich. A palm of grapes contains anywhere between sixty and one hundred calories.

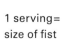

1 serving=
size of fist

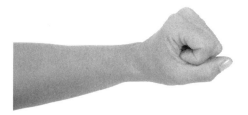

Dairy: Two hundred calories from this group will likely come from milk (try 2 percent or skim; they are lower in fat and have more nutrients), cheese, or yogurt. An eight-ounce glass of milk contains about a hundred calories, as does a thumb of cheese, a small yogurt cup, a small pudding cup, or a cup (eight ounces) of soy milk.

Most women do not consume the one thousand to twelve hundred milligrams of calcium needed in a day, so it's always good to be taking a multivitamin. If you're consuming two dairy servings with this plan, you are getting anywhere from six hundred to eight hundred milligrams of calcium.

1 serving=
size of fist

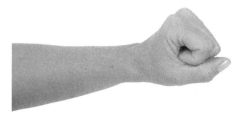

Lindsay's Rule of Thumb

Cheese is one of the exceptions to the palm method. Instead of using your palm to measure a correct portion of cheese, use your thumb. One thumb-size chunk of cheese equals one palm.

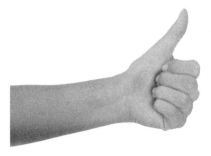

1 serving=
size of thumb

Protein: Your three servings of protein will provide you with between three hundred and six hundred calories. Ideally, you will get some protein from other sources besides red meat. If you do choose red meat, opt for leaner cuts. Generally, any loin cut of meat is leaner than other cuts. Loin contains approximately two hundred calories in a three-ounce portion. Less lean cuts contain about three hundred calories per three ounces. Here are some calorie equivalents for other protein sources. Each of these is equal to approximately 150 calories:

1 cup of beans
¾ cup of cottage cheese
1 palm of nuts
¾ cup of 2 percent shredded cheese
2 tablespoons of peanut butter
15 small shrimp
3 medium or 2 large eggs
1 palm of chicken, pork, or fish

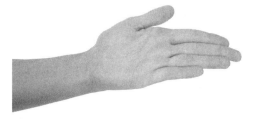

1 serving=
palm of hand

Fat: The smallest amount of calories of any group should come from fat. The one hundred calories you should consume can come from lots of sources, but remember what I've said about good, bad, and worse fats. Many types of nuts are a source of good protein, but mostly when they are eaten raw or dry roasted. One tablespoon of extra-virgin olive equals approximately one hundred calories, as does half of an avocado, one tablespoon of mayonnaise, one tablespoon of olive oil and vinegar salad dressing, and eight canned or bottled olives.

1 serving=
size of thumb

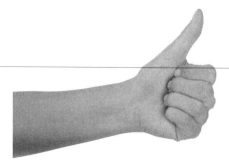

Carbs/Grains/Starches: I mentioned earlier the importance of eating whole grains. Don't be deceived by seven-grain or nine-grain; they are often not whole grains. Look for the word *whole* in the ingredients list when deciding what to consume to get to your three hundred calories for this group. One starch equals one hundred calories, the caloric equivalent of a half cup of pasta, potatoes, or rice; two slices of whole-wheat bread; half of a whole-wheat pita; or a small baked white potato.

1 serving=
cup of hand

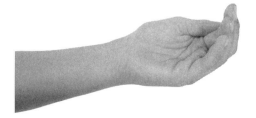

FAT-BURNING FOODS,
OR HIGH-VOLUME FOODS

There's a lot of debate about whether or not certain foods actually help your body to burn fat. I'm not going to spend a lot of time on the debate, but I will say this: I call these foods high-volume foods, because they make you feel fuller sooner and they have a low calorie content, which also makes them ideal to eat. For a list of these foods, go to momswhothink.com/diet-and-nutrition/fat-burning-foods.html. Among those listed are apples, beans, berries, tofu, spinach, and whole grains. No surprises there, but the list also includes foods such as pasta, kiwi, chicken, turkey, and mustard—especially the hot Asian varieties. I don't think researchers have definitively identified how these foods work to get your body to burn fat stores, but they are all nutrient rich, high-volume foods, so you certainly won't go wrong eating any of them.

Sugar Detox

Anytime you fall off the wagon, this is a good tool to get you back on. Eliminate all simple sugars for three days and replace them with fruits and vegetables. You'll be back on track and not craving sugary stuff!

One of the things you have to learn is to feel full with your stomach and not with your eyes. If I were to put a small serving of your favorite fast-food french fries in front of you, I bet you would eat less than if I had put a large portion in front of you. With a large portion, you would feel full, but your eyes would tell you there's more there. The clean plate club was a good idea when you were a kid and you were being encouraged to eat all your veggies, but that habit may have had a bad long-term effect on you. I believe in clean plates, but as I mentioned above, your plate should start with high-bulk vegetables covering half of it.

SLIM CHANCES

These are things we all do as moms, but there's a slim chance that it's helping you reach your goal!

You eat off your children's plates. The moms of Moms Into Fitness call it a BLT: a bite, lick, or taste. You can consume three hundred to four hundred calories without realizing it. You'll need to exercise thirty extra minutes to get rid of these calories.

You eat too quickly. It takes twenty minutes to register fullness. Eat slowly, and drink one cup, or eight ounces, of water before diving into your meal and one cup, or eight ounces, during your meal. And always sit down while eating.

You eat dinner twice. You eat dinner with your children at five o'clock and again with your partner at seven. Try to fulfill your servings of vegetables (two and a half cups daily) while eating with your children, and eat the remainder of dinner with your partner. And remember, your body does not care what time you consume calories; it only cares if you consume too many calories!

You eat because you're drained. If you consume fewer than a thousand calories a day, you do need to eat for more energy. But in most cases, only exercise and sleep will help get you out of your slump.

You eat everything out of a box or bag. More than likely the foods that come from a box or bag have hydrogenated oils and empty calories. Think ahead of time and pack fruits and veggies for the car ride or running out the door. These provide fullness, nutrients, and fiber.

SNACKS

Here are some low-fat snacks both you and your children will enjoy. (These are for your older children—obviously not the one you just had! Some are choking hazards for young children.)

Hot chocolate and marshmallows (made at home with skim milk)
Strawberries dipped in chocolate pudding
Cottage cheese mixed with sliced peaches
Small pizzas: use a cookie cutter to cut store-bought pizza dough; pile with pizza sauce and shredded cheese)
Veggie pizza: next time you make spinach, puree some and put it in your pizza sauce
Cinnamon and sugar toast with milk
Tortilla roll-ups: layer ham and cheese on a flour tortilla, roll up, and cut into small pieces
Vanilla pudding with crumbled low-fat cookies
Zucchini sticks: lightly coat slices of zucchini with bread crumbs, bake, and serve with pizza sauce

The Fitness Program

Eating right is only one part of the best choice you can make to shed those pounds and inches. Exercise is the other important component of feeling good and looking good. I'm all about doing things efficiently and multitasking, and I know you don't have hours a day to work out. That's why my program calls for you to exercise for thirty to fifty-five minutes five times a week, with the fifteen-minute express stroller workout option. How can you get results when you used to spend up to an hour or an hour and a half every day in the gym? You can burn just as many calories—sometimes more—if you interval train for those thirty minutes as opposed to walking (or jogging) at a constant pace. And if you can give 100 percent in that thirty minutes, you're cooking like gas!

Will I ever fit back into a bikini? Sure! Follow my exercise program by working your TA and PF. Then use my nutrition tricks to keep your calories within the range you calculated on page 254. No gimmicks, just pure science. So just strolling with your stroller won't make you lose weight fast—to get your body back into a bikini we need to bump it up! This means you need to get into your fat-burning zone. And without getting into too much detail (I know you're short on time), we're going to keep you breathing hard with this workout. Overall you should be close to fatigue during your last few repetitions, and you should be breathless during the cardio portions. It's time to throw out the pregnancy eating as well as the pregnancy workout rules. That is, unless you are pregnant again. And if you're breast-feeding, you're still eating like you did while pregnant.

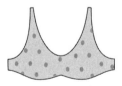

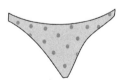

The Stroller 10 Workout

Frequency:

Monday: Stroller 10 (work out inside if the weather is bad)
Tuesday: Cardio A, Cardio B, or Cardio C
Wednesday: Stroller 10
Thursday: Cardio A, Cardio B, Cardio C, or REST
Friday: Stroller 10 or my *Postnatal Boot Camp* DVD (if you own this DVD you
    can throw it into the schedule by using the create-a-workout and tailoring
    your workout to the time you have available)

Duration: 30–45 minutes

You can do it on the sidewalk in your neighborhood or at your local park. (And, of course, if you have time, I *never* discourage more cardio—running, walking, swimming, hiking, kickboxing, and so on.) You probably won't be able to dedicate five days to exercise every week. All I ask is that you try! But I have built in a fifteen-minute express stroller workout to replace the Stroller 10 on Monday, Wednesday, and Friday.

    Do not use the Stroller 10 workout outside if it's too hot, too cold, raining, or plain old bad weather! Instead, work out inside—each stroller exercise transforms to an exercise in the comfort of your own home, and with your baby! I call it the "inside workout"; it's on page 277.

    Rules: Lock your stroller's wheels and wrap the stroller leash around a non-moving part of your body (like your arm when you do curtsies). Exercise in a safe area (a park or a neighborhood during daylight), watch the weather, and use the "inside workout" if needed. Also use sunblock on yourself and the kids. You can stop in the shade to perform the ten exercises if you like.

    Equipment needed: Bring a towel or mat; you will be getting on your hands and knees. You'll also need an exercise band or hand weights, which you can purchase at just about any discount department store, such as Target or Walmart. Finally, bring whatever you need to keep your child happy and healthy while you finish the workout.

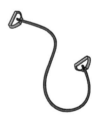

Exercise bands
for stroller exercises

CARDIO OPTIONS A, B, AND C FOR TUESDAY AND THURSDAY

A. 30 minutes: Alternate walking 2 minutes and jogging 2 minutes for a total of 30 minutes. For a more advanced workout, jog 2 minutes and run 2 minutes. (Run is about 15–20 percent faster than jog. Hate jogging? Walk and use some hills).

B. 20–30 minutes: Use a stroller pedometer to walk or jog 2.5 miles. Each week try to decrease the time you accomplish your 2.5 miles

C. 26 minutes (inside): Use my *Postnatal Boot Camp* DVD—you can mix and match the short segments to make a cardio workout you have time for! Try the 3-minute warm-up, 10-minute Kardio Kickboxing, 10-minute Just Cardio, and 3-minute cooldown (add Kardio Kickboxing again after Just Cardio for an extra calorie burn!).

A FEW MORE WORDS ON STROLLERS

Some doctors recommend that you avoid using a jogging stroller until your child is four to six months of age, but these days you can put the car seat into a lot of jogging strollers. Your baby does not have a lot of head control, and a car seat is more secure. Some strollers work as both a jogging and an everyday stroller. Either way, your baby should be able to support his or her head without a car seat. But if you are walking or jogging with a regular stroller and car seat, please place a towel around baby's head to keep it supported.

If you are going to use a jogging stroller, there are two main types: all terrain and regular. The main difference is that the front wheel swivels on the all terrain. Both have rubber wheels about sixteen inches in diameter. No matter

Do You Have More Than One Child for the Stroller?

The more weight in your stroller, the bigger the challenge for your body, and the better results! Of course, you may not be able to follow the jogging intervals as well, but try it! I'll never forget Mindy from my stroller class. She had eight-month-old triplets and a seven-year-old son, who would walk beside her. What a workout—physically *and* mentally!

which one you purchase, make sure it has a five-point harness and that it safely fits your child. I recommend that you buy one that is easy to fold up, lightweight, and the right height for you. Go to the store and try a few before buying!

As always, you must warm up before exercising. In the stroller exercises you will walk for five minutes prior to the beginning of the workout.

Always lock your stroller when you stop to do any of the exercises below!

You will notice you are not using the stroller in all the exercises. If you did, you would isolate the lower body.

Be cautious—especially on the frog jumps—not to tip your stroller. Only use the stroller bar to keep it a few feet in front of you, not to hold your balance!

Remember all the exercises basics—exhale on the effort, engage your core (PF and TA), and maintain good posture throughout! Refer to page 82 for the illustration on finding your TA and activating it!

I Want to Reduce My Hips!

Blood circulates all over your body, right? You have water all over your body, right? You have fat all over your body, right? Well, you don't refer to the blood in your belly as "belly blood" that stays in your belly . . . and you cannot refer to the fat on your belly as "belly fat." Fat will be reduced all over your body when you exercise; there is no such thing as spot reduction.

Repetitions: Perform 20 of each exercise.

1. **Walking ab lunge:** Stand with your feet shoulder-width apart and hold on to the stroller. Step into a lunge by stepping forward about three feet with one leg. Flex the opposite knee so that your back leg is approximately six inches off the ground. Return to standing position and bring your back leg into a knee lift. Now lunge forward with the lifted knee. Each time your right leg goes forward counts as one repetition.

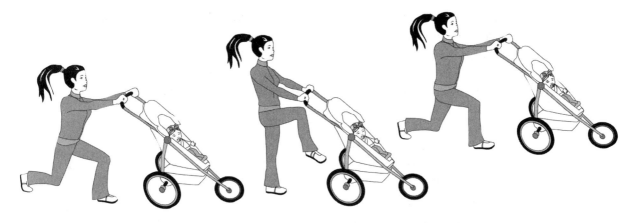

Walking ab lunge

2. **Squat and twist:** Use the exercise band. Lock your stroller to your side and place the middle of the band under your right foot, about one foot away from your left foot. Grab both handles of the band and squat. Twist by leading with your straight arms to the left. Return to starting position. After 20 repetitions, switch sides. An easy modification is to grab only one handle of the band.

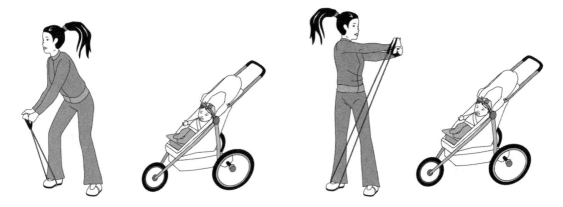

Squat and twist

Using a weight instead of an exercise band?

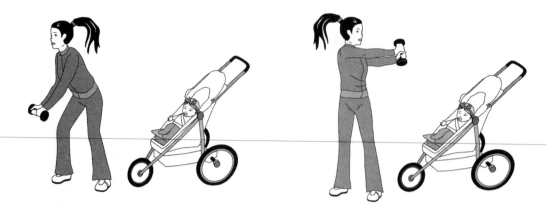

Squat and twist with weight

3. **Single-arm triceps extension:** Use the exercise band. Lock your stroller to your side. Place the middle of the band under your right foot and grab one handle with your right hand. Raise your arm straight up alongside your ear with your palm facing your head. Bend and extend your elbow. After 20 repetitions, switch arms.

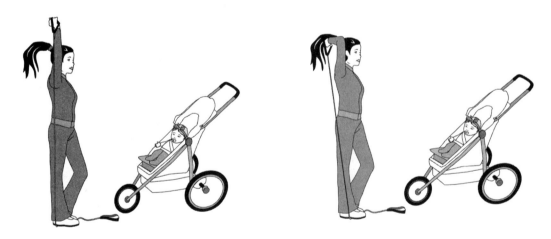

Single-arm triceps extension

Using a weight instead of an exercise band?

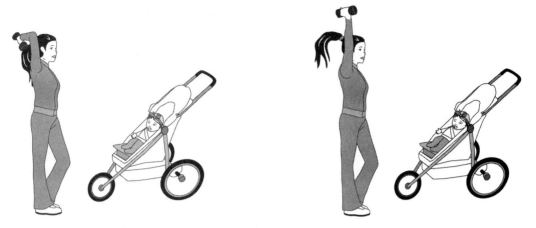

Single-arm triceps extension, with weight

4. **Curtsy to abduct:** Hold on to the stroller. With your feet twelve to eighteen inches apart, perform a curtsy and then abduct your leg: Lift it to the outside about thirty inches from your other foot. After 20 repetitions, switch legs.

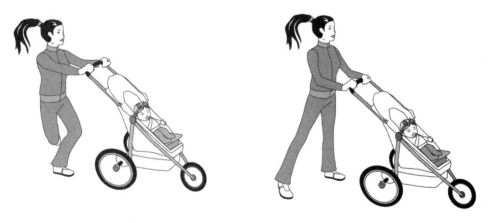

Curtsy to abduct

5. **Rotating "girl" push-up:** Kneel down on all fours with your hands directly under your shoulders in a modified plank. Raise one hand and twist your torso so that your arm is perpendicular to the ground. Return to the modified plank and raise your other hand to the other side. When you are feeling strong enough, do a push-up in modified plank before raising your hand to the other side. Be sure to lock the stroller at your side.

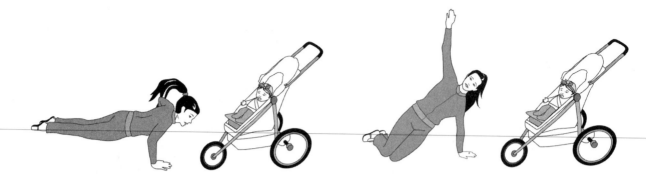

Rotating "girl" push-up

6. **Plié to soccer sweep:** Hold on to the stroller. Stand with your feet at least two feet apart and your toes pointed outward forty-five degrees or more. While keeping your back straight, bend both knees. As you return to starting position, sweep your leg in front of you as if you were kicking a soccer ball. Do twenty reps on one leg, then switch.

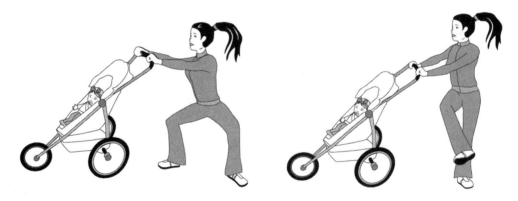

Plié to soccer sweep

7. **Frog jumps:** Stand with your feet shoulder-width apart and your hands on the stroller's bar. Bend your knees so that you are in a shallow squat (knees bent no more than sixty degrees). Hold that position briefly before jumping up as high as you can. Be sure to point your toes on the jump. Do *not* push down on the stroller.

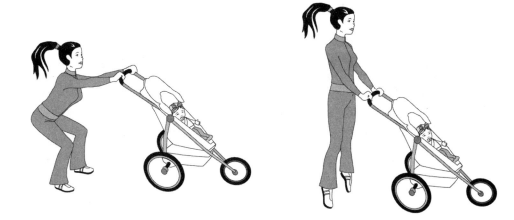

Frog jumps

8. **Plank abductions:** Lock the stroller off to your side. Begin on all fours with your shoulders directly above your hands. Move into the plank position. Keep your elbows soft. Abduct your left leg, bring it back to center, then abduct your right leg. As you move each leg, don't drop the opposite hip; keep it parallel to the ground.

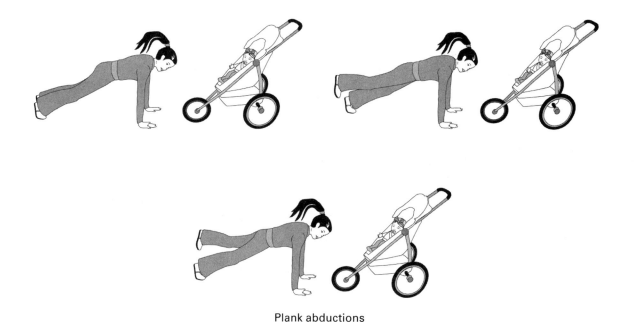

Plank abductions

9. **Single-leg squat and press:** Use the exercise band. Lock the stroller to your side. Place the middle of the band under your left foot and put all of your weight on that foot while leaving your right toe on the ground. Grasp one handle of the band with your left hand and bring it to shoulder height. Squat with your right leg while raising your arm above your head. Return to starting position. Do 20 reps on one leg, then switch.

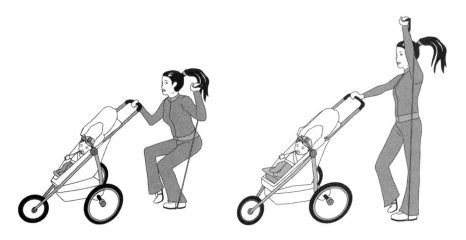

Single-leg squat and press

Using a weight instead of an exercise band?

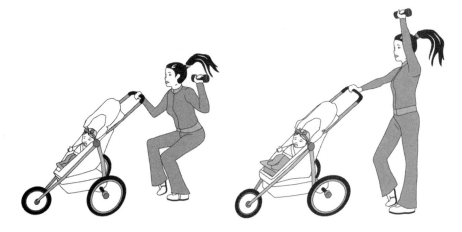

Single-leg squat and press, with weight

10. Screamers: Hold on to your stroller. Bend forward at the hips in a slight lunge position. Keeping your weight on your front leg, bend that leg and touch the other toe two feet behind you. Bring the back leg to your chest. Do 20 reps on one leg, then switch. This is a fast-moving exercise.

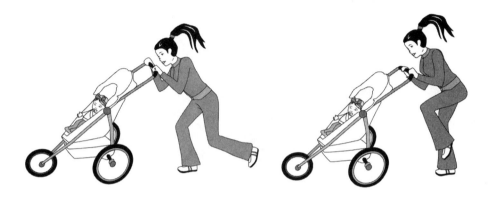

Screamers

We don't want to forget about targeting your core, so you should always start or conclude the Stroller 10 with a sequence of five exercises I call the Ab 5. You activated your core throughout the Stroller 10 and even used it in most of the exercises. Now do the Ab 5—you can do this at home, but I recommend doing it while you're out. We all find excuses to not exercise when we get home—don't let the important core work get away from you!

Remember to stretch your hip flexors and quads before doing any abdominal work.

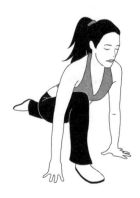

The Ab 5

1. 30 boomerangs
2. 20 seals
3. Hold asymmetrical push-up position 1 minute
4. 40 bicycles
5. 2 elbow taps

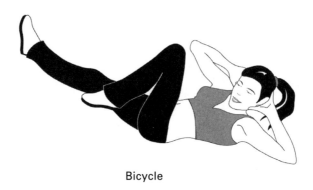

Bicycle

You did four of these in the CFS method; we added the bicycles this time around. Go to page 205 for a refresher. Even on a day you cannot possibly fit anything in, even the Express Stroller Workout (on page 279), fit this in!

CORE BABY

When you hold your baby on your hip, you are probably sticking your hip out to the side to create a platform for baby to sit. When you do that, make sure you don't stick out your abs! Remember core activation (if you need a reminder, go to page 92).

Inside Workout

Perform the same workout with your stroller inside the house. But you will replace the cardio blast with the cardio block below. Of course, if you don't want to use the stroller, place your baby in a bouncy seat or other safe place and he or she can watch you work out.

Cardio Block

1 minute of jumping jacks
1 minute of mountain climbers (from the floor in a plank position, "run" your knees in and out)

OR

2 minutes of walking or running up and down the stairs inside your house

> If you are back to getting your periods, know that your hormones fluctuate during your cycle, which can make you either more or less hungry. But you are in charge of what goes in your mouth, even if your hormones are bossing you around!

The Schedule: Six-Week Plan

Now that you know what the Stroller 10 exercises are like, here is the schedule you will follow for the next six weeks. The Monday through Friday breakdown is on page 266.

WEEKS 1 AND 2 (STROLLER 10 WORKOUT: BEGINNERS: 30 MINUTES; VETERANS: 40 MINUTES; MONDAY, WEDNESDAY, FRIDAY)

Warm-up: 3-minute walk

Beginners and veterans: 20 reps each:

1. Walking ab lunge
   a. Cardio blast: Beginners: walk 1 minute, jog 1 minute. Veterans: jog 1½ minutes, walk 30 seconds.

If you are not comfortable jogging, please replace with a speed walk, or even a walk up a hill for a better calorie burn.

---

2. Squat and twist w/band
3. Single arm triceps extension w/band
   a. Cardio blast
4. Curtsy to abduct
5. Rotating girl push-ups or real push-ups
   a. Cardio blast
6. Plié to soccer sweep
7. Frog jumps
   a. Cardio blast
8. Plank abductions
9. Single leg squat and press w/band
   a. Cardio blast
10. Screamers

Veterans: You will then repeat the Stroller 10 when you get home, with no cardio blasts. Do this after completing the Ab 5.

Cooldown: Walk 1–2 minutes.

Ab 5 outside or when you get home

Post-pregnancy stretches (page 208)

EXPRESS STROLLER WORKOUT

This workout can be done inside or outside, with or without your stroller.

Stroller 10: Perform 20 repetitions of each of the 10 toning exercises (rest in between if needed)

Ab 5

Jump Without Peeing on Yourself!

You've trained your pelvic floor already—now put it to the test. Do Kegels while you jump-rope. (If you're using the inside workout, you will be doing jumping jacks.)

If you are a jogger, replace the walk with a jog and the jog with a run (10 to 20 percent faster than your comfortable jog). You'll notice you will get faster and faster!

WEEKS 3 AND 4 (50 MINUTES)

Beginners: We are really bumping it up this week, so please listen to your body and stop when you need to, even if you cut the workout short. And, of course, break when you need to.

The last thing I want is for you to get frustrated with this workout! So please use this as your warning: It will be somewhat difficult, and you may want to quit. But next week it will be a lot easier.

Warm-up: 3-minute walk

Beginners: 2 sets of 12 repetitions

Veterans: 2 sets of 15 repetitions (20-second rest between sets)

1. Walking ab lunge
   a. Cardio blast: Beginners: walk 1 minute, jog 1 minute. Veterans: jog 1½ minutes, run 30 seconds.

> If you are not comfortable jogging, please replace with a speed walk, or even a walk up a hill for a better calorie burn.

2. Squat and twist w/band
3. Single-arm triceps extension w/band
   a. Cardio blast
4. Curtsy to abduct
5. Rotating girl push-ups or real push-ups
   a. Cardio blast
6. Plié to soccer sweep
7. Frog jumps
   a. Cardio blast
8. Plank abductions
9. Single-leg squat and press with band
   a. Cardio blast
10. Screamers

Cooldown: Walk 1–2 minutes.
Ab 5 outside or when you get home
Post-pregnancy stretches (page 208)

> Veterans, your running pace should be 15–20 percent faster than your jog.

WEEKS 5 AND 6 (55 MINUTES)

You will be doing the Ab 5 after the warm-up and before the cooldown.

Perform all 10 exercises with 2 minutes of jogging between each or use Cadio Blast.

Warm-up: 3-minute walk

Ab 5

Beginners: 2 sets of 15 repetitions (20-second rest between sets)

Veterans: 2 sets of 18 repetitions (20-second rest between sets)

1. Walking ab lunge
   a. Cardio blast: Beginners: walk 30 seconds, jog 1½ minutes. Veterans: jog 1 minute, run 1 minute.

> If you are not comfortable jogging, please replace with a speed walk, or even a walk up a hill for a better calorie burn.

2. Squat and twist w/band
3. Single-arm triceps extension w/band
   a. Cardio blast
4. Curtsy to abduct
5. Rotating girl push-ups or real push-ups
   a. Cardio blast
6. Plié to soccer sweep
7. Frog jumps
   a. Cardio blast
8. Plank abductions
9. Single-leg squat and press with band
   a. Cardio blast
10. Screamers

Cooldown: 2 minute walk

Ab 5 (again) outside or when you get home

Post-pregnancy stretches (page 208)

Are you wide awake at five a.m. after feeding the baby? Go ahead and get out of bed and start your workout outside *without* the stroller (as long as your partner is home to take care of the baby/kids). I love doing this. Or I will set a jug of water and mat outside my front door, then jog a lap around the block, stop in my driveway for 20 push-ups, 20 screamers, and an Ab 5, and repeat the whole sequence for a total of 3 times.

WEEK 7 AND BEYOND

Why does the workout change every few weeks? The reason is your body gets used to doing the same exercises, and the inevitable plateau arrives at your doorstep. To prevent this slump, I also created workout downloads. There is a new workout every thirty days that you can download directly to your computer for five dollars a month from momsintofitness.com/dvds/downloads.

Remember how important variety of exercise is! I want to provide you with many ways to lose weight, so whether you're doing a kickboxing class, training for a triathlon, walking at the park, or exercising with your baby, get something in five days a week. My rule? Three of those days must be intense training. The American College of Sports Medicine recently had a study that determined that short, intense bouts of exercise are best. What does that mean for you? Well, less time, but it also means hard work while you're committed to that ten, twenty, or thirty minutes. Intense training is the Stroller 10 workout, any of my DVDs, and so on. In one thirty-minute stroller workout you will burn between three hundred and four hundred calories. In a forty-five-minute stroller workout you will burn about five hundred calories.

Are you up for the challenge?

You can use the maintenance workout here or start something different. Increase your weights to rev up that metabolism. Your body needs a change every now and again, so try something new!

Exercise is so crucial to weight loss and maintenance. Most of us consume more calories than we should, and it's a lot easier to add something to our lives (exercise) than it is to take something away (excess food). That's just human nature. There are a lot of people out there who like exercise and physical activity (I'm one!), but that's not true of everybody. I do think that once you get past the initial stages of discomfort and unfamiliarity you will, like nearly every one of my clients, develop an appreciation for exercise—especially when you see how it is benefiting you.

I do this for a living, so it's a bit easier for me. Sure, I have to say no (most of the time) to a peanut butter cookie at the mall as my daughter smiles happily with crumbs all over her face. And I have to say no to the yummy snacks that stare at me after the kids have gone to bed, and to finishing off the enormous portion of fries that came with my club sandwich. But know that every mom out there is feeling the same and trying to tackle daily reminders of the need to lose weight. I want you to do this workout plan so you feel better about yourself.

Of course, there are days I don't want to work out, but then I just remember how I feel after even ten minutes of doing something small. My mood improves 100 percent. So just do it, just for the mood boost—your family will appreciate it! The next time you tell yourself you just don't want to do it use the five-minute rule.

Rule #9: Just begin the workout, and if after five minutes you want to be done, be done. More than likely you will want to continue!

Warm-up: 3-minute walk

Ab 5 at the beginning of this workout and again at the end, after the warm-up and the cooldown: Perform 1 minute of each exercise: flight, plank clock, elbow taps, butterfly crunch with pelvic tilt and Kegel, bicycle.

If you don't remember how to do these core exercises, flip to Part II; you've done them before, and you've been doing the bicycle for the past six weeks.

20 reps each:

1. Walking ab lunge
2. Squat and twist w/band
3. Single arm triceps extension w/band
4. Curtsy to abduct (do 20 before switching sides)
5. Rotating girl push-ups or real push-ups

Beginners: 2-minute walk, 2-minute jog, sprint for 50 steps, repeat from walk

Veterans: 2-minute jog, 2-minute run, sprint for 50 steps, repeat from jog
Repeat exercises 1–5.

6. Plié to soccer sweep
7. Frog jumps
8. Plank abductions
9. Single-leg squat and press w/band
10. Screamers (do 20 before switching sides)

Repeat exercises 6–10.

> Remember, you can always replace the jog with speed walking up a hill.

Ab 5 (again) outside or when you get home
Post-pregnancy stretches (page 208)

> Keep yourself and your child well hydrated while outside.

Cellulite

Since fitness is in the eye of the beholder, let's talk about a certain genetic disadvantage women have to overcome: cellulite.

With all the misconceptions about cellulite remedies—creams, theories, dissolves, wraps, and the like—I thought I could clear up a few things for you. First and foremost, cellulite is plain old fat. And the only way to get rid of it without surgery is through nutrition and exercise (mostly exercise).

I could stop here and say that's all you need to know, but I will go into a little more detail. The more muscle you have, the smoother you can look. Why do some fit women still have cellulite? Women's fat cells are separated into honeycomb-like compartments. Fat can push through these honeycombs and create the cottage cheese effect. Your genetics determines where and how many fat cells you have. So why don't men seem to have cellulite like women? The answer lies in male genetics. They are blessed with streamlined connective tissue instead of honeycombs.

You can minimize the appearance of cellulite through exercise. First, exercise regularly to decrease the odds of even developing cellulite. *But*, if you already have it, you can diminish the dimpled look with a regular combination of toning and cardio. The best (and easiest) way to achieve this is through interval training. Overall toning is the most important component of losing the dimples. And muscle boosts your metabolism, which helps you burn the fat!

Keep in mind nutritional decisions are also very important in fat loss and cellulite minimization.

Now, you can't do anything about the past or your genetics, but you can do a lot about your future. As I'll talk about a lot more in the pages ahead, the best thing you can do is incorporate a consistent workout program that includes toning and cardio three to five times a week, and you will see significant cellulite reduction results within six to eight weeks.

A few words about those creams, wraps and surgery to reduce cellulite: No cream applied to the skin can penetrate and rearrange the fat cells beneath the surface. You can compress fat, and this is why some methods seem to work—temporarily. Wraps only work for about twenty-four to seventy-two hours. Liposuction permanently removes fat cells, but if more than 10 percent of weight is gained afterward, old fat cells simply get bigger.

As we women get older, our skin gets a little thinner. So even a little bit of cellulite will show through. Combine that with our metabolism getting a little slower as we age, and our fat production increases. Combat this and get on

---

Three of the top questions I receive from moms are a) Should I get a tummy tuck? b) Should I get liposuction? and c) How do I get rid of my loose skin?

And here's my answer:

If you can answer the first two questions with 100 percent confidence, then plastic surgery may be for you. Have you been consistent with your exercise (emphasizing toning) and nutrition for at least a year? Do you feel you have done everything in your power without excuses to achieve the body you have always wanted? If you answer no, then the answer to the questions above is *no*.

I want to hear from you! Chat with me on Facebook (facebook.com/momsintofitness) or though my blog. And I'd love to hear through our casting calls how you got your body back. Just visit momsintofitness.com!

the exercise train! Seriously, take the opportunity to be proactive and prevent excess cellulite!

1 pound LEAN MUSCLE vs. 1 pound FAT TISSUE

Don't believe the myth: Muscle doesn't necessarily make you bulkier or cause the numbers on the scale to shoot up. In fact, if you compare a pound of muscle and a pound of fat, it's easy to see why building muscle is so important to get your body into shape. Fat tissue is not exactly attractive. Fat is ugly and undefined, while muscle is smooth and takes up less space. Fat actually makes your waistline bigger by just being fat, as it takes up more space than muscle. Most of us want to get rid of the fat to get fit, but it's important to remember that building muscle will give you the lean, toned physique you want.

Stay away from diet pills and anything else that promises quick results—they're gimmicks. You *have* to eat well and exercise to lose weight and improve your health. That's all I have to say about diet pills, which somehow gross more money than any fitness DVD.

Staying in Balance

Your mental and emotional health are just as important as your physical health. Being a mom, it's important to try and balance all three—and the best part is exercise can help you achieve the balance!

What If You Are Gaining Weight?

Do weekly weigh-ins and measurements (measure biceps at biggest part, bust at biggest part, one inch above waist, one inch below waist, biggest part around hips, and biggest part around thigh—measure the same side, right or left, every time).

- If you gained 2 pounds or an overall 1–2 inches, it's time to start watching it.

- If you gained 4 pounds or an overall 3–4 inches, it's time to add some extra cardio workouts.
- If you gained 6 or more pounds at any point, remember that consistent workouts help you maintain your weight.

You *must* food-journal and make sure you are eating calories within your BMR.

Do you still have 10, 20, or 80 pounds to go? It's time to switch up the workout. Your goal should be 4 to 6 pounds a month for a 10- to 20-pound weight loss and 6 to 10 pounds a month for a 30- to 80-pound weight loss. Remember, if you have thirty minutes out of 1,440 in a day, you can do it! And be honest with yourself—are you making a 100 percent effort to achieve your goal? Or are you sedentary some days?

If you have not lost your baby weight by nine months post-delivery and didn't gain more than forty or fifty pounds you are a) simply eating too much; or b) not exercising enough (as long as you don't have diabetes, hypothyroidism, PPD, etc.).

Now that I have my body where I want it, I need to do interval training only twice a week and interval cardio once a week. I really enjoy getting my cardio with a jogging stroller and interval run. And I always do my *Boot Camp*

SKINNY PEOPLE TRICKS

Here are a few ideas you can try that have been proven winners for people who intelligently manage their weight:

- Use small bowls and plates to trick your eyes.
- Side items, such as a baked potato, can make a filling meal.
- Never eat pasta out of a bowl; use a plate instead.
- If it's not good, stop eating! Why indulge in something you dislike? Save the calories.
- If you like candy, cut yourself off after 150 calories (about one handful).
- When you feel full, throw out or package the remaining food immediately. I have even seen women pour sugar on their hamburger once they have had half of it.

- Drink one glass (eight ounces) of water before a meal and one glass of water during the meal.
- Use the palm of your hand as a size guide for proteins.
- Eat ice cream out of a cone instead of a bowl.
- Put in retainers or tooth-whitening trays at your "pitfall" time, or when you tend to eat the most. For most moms, that is after the kids go to bed. Brush your teeth and cut yourself off.
- Thin-crust pizza, never thick-crust.
- Mustard instead of mayo on sandwiches.
- Pass on the bread basket! Not because bread is bad, but because you can easily consume four hundred calories with a roll or two before you've even had dinner. And for a 5'4" woman who weighs about 140 pounds, that's a quarter of the calories for the day!
- Schedule your workout during your "witching hour."

We tend to eat with our eyes and not register fullness. These tricks can help you eat less and still feel full.

2 DVD for some ten-minute toning. So down the road you might be able to decrease the frequency of your workouts. (But you'll have to increase intensity to keep challenging that new body!)

Why Do My Clothes Fit a Bit Too Tight?

The cold, hard truth from a personal trainer: You need to burn more calories than you consume.

- You absolutely cannot eat the amount of food you would like (sorry).
- Dessert is a habit; habits can be broken.
- Out of sight, out of mind! Remove the M&M's from your desk or your pantry.
- Ordering pizza for dinner? Sure, but stay away from pepperoni, sausage, and cheese-filled crust. Oh, and you don't need the extra cheesy bread.

- Finally, can you go to bed saying to yourself, "I feel good about the food choices I made today"? If you can, give yourself a pat on the back!

Be *very* aware of what you are putting in your mouth. Sounds easy, right? Are you guilty of grabbing a yummy cheddar fish cracker every time you get a snack out for the kids? Guilty of grabbing a chocolate kiss out of the office candy jar? Guilty of eating the leftovers on your kids' plates?

If any of this sounds familiar, it is probably the reason you cannot lose the inevitable last five or ten pounds. Think exercise is impossible with your hectic schedule? Just try it for five minutes a day—it can be quite rejuvenating!

CONCLUSION

ongratulations! You've reached the end of the book. Of course, that doesn't necessarily mean that you're done with the work. In the few pages before this you saw what you need to do to continue. Remember, variety is the spice of life, which is so true for your workouts. Spice them up and have fun! I hope there are a few sweat stains on these pages, even if some of those stains are from tears of adjusting to motherhood—from the satisfaction you've experienced in seeing all of your hard work pay off.

I know from experience that being a mom is a lot of hard work, and that work is also the most rewarding thing you've ever done. I hope you feel the same way about your fitness program. I'm sure there have been a few ups and downs—and not just the ones you experienced while doing crunches or squats—but that's all a part of the journey. Incorporating fitness into your daily routine is an important part of taking care of you. It's the best mood stabilizer there is—you don't want your partner dangling running shoes in front of you every day! So if for no other reason you joined in this fitness program, remember: You can't take good care of your family if you don't take good care of yourself.

I'm so happy that I could share with you my experiences and insights, and I truly hope they have been beneficial. Please know that I'm right there along with you, putting in the effort and measuring the results just as you are. Let's do this together, and let's be sure to celebrate along the way!

APPENDIX A

Sample 7-Day Menu for Part III

Once again, I am not going to give you a grocery list of items you have to eat. What I've listed below is a sample menu that will keep you within the BMR range of eleven hundred to sixteen hundred calories. As moms, we need to be able to change our schedule at the drop of a hat. Look at one day, or look at all seven days if you need more guidance.

I love to cook, but I am not a chef by any means! What you will find below are tried-and-true easy recipes by moms like you. They will keep you in your calorie budget and allow you to get all the food groups we discussed earlier. Pay attention to the servings, as most of the recipes are divided when you make the meal. You can easily substitute—you're a mom and every day is different and busy. But try to plan ahead.

You will also see that there are a few leftovers in the sample menu. This is to make it easier on you! Although my husband complains when we have leftovers, the plan below tosses the ingredients together in a different mix so he'll never know. This is what I use in my household, and it works. Each serving is 1 *adult* serving, since you probably have to make something different for the kids (I am talking about older kids, not the baby you just had). And, well, I know kids are the pickiest! Although they will enjoy the taco soup.

DAY 1

Recipes are provided below.

Breakfast: Raspberry smoothie
Snack: 1 piece fruit
Lunch: 1 Mediterranean pita pizza
Snack: 1 serving black bean dip
Dinner: 1 grocery store rotisserie chicken (yields 8 servings without dark meat) and 1 package broccoli woccoli (found in the produce section—follow directions for steaming) topped with 1 tablespoon olive oil, salt, and pepper. Have as many steamed vegetables as you like, but stick to about 2 palm-size servings of rotisserie chicken.

DAY 2

Breakfast: 1 piece fruit and 1 instant oatmeal (the flavored packets are just as nutritious)
Snack: ½ Mediterranean pita pizza (leftover)
Lunch: 1 serving Mexican soup
Snack: 6 oz yogurt
Dinner: 1 serving sweet and sour shrimp kebab and 1 piece of fruit

DAY 3

Breakfast: 1 cup grapes and 2 pieces whole-wheat toast
Snack: 6 oz yogurt
Lunch: Make 2 lettuce wraps with leftover rotisserie chicken
Snack: Shrimp cocktail (6–12 medium cooked shrimp and 2 tablespoons cocktail sauce) or 2 servings tossed apple salad
Dinner: 1–2 soft beef tacos, optional side salad with veggies and a few tablespoons olive-oil-based dressing

DAY 4

Breakfast: 1 8 oz drinkable yogurt and an apple

Snack: Veggies and 2–3 tablespoons hummus

Lunch: 1 serving Mexican soup. In a hurry? Make a homemade grilled cheese, spinach, and tomato sandwich with a side of steamed vegetables (your choice) or Campbell's tomato Soup at Hand.

Snack: 1 cup grapes or raspberries

Dinner: 1–2 servings 6-ingredient Mexican soup (leftover)

DAY 5

Breakfast: 1 English muffin melt

Snack: 1 serving trail mix

Lunch: 1 serving raspberry salad

Snack: 1 serving zucchini stix

Dinner: 1–2 servings stuffed green pepper soup

DAY 6

Breakfast: 1 instant oatmeal made with skim milk

Snack: Raspberry parfait or chocolate-covered strawberries

Lunch: 1 serving tuna salad with toasted pita

Snack: ½ serving raspberry salad (leftover)

Dinner: 1 serving meatless chili with a handful of turtilla chips

DAY 7

Breakfast: 1 egg pita and ½ cup raspberries

Snack: 1 cup grapes

Lunch: 2 servings Tex-Mex salad

Snack: ½ cup meatless chili (leftover)

Dinner: 1 serving pork chop dinner

Optional calorie-free or low-calorie dessert:

- Hot tea (my personal favorite is vanilla almond) is the best dessert ever, and guilt-free!
- Low-fat homemade hot cocoa
- Fresh fruit: 1 piece or ½ cup berries

Add a cup of skim milk to any meal (just not *every* meal)!

APPENDIX B

Sample Recipes

I've histed recipes from my 7-day sample menu, as well as a few recipes to create your own menu!

QUICK-PREP, LOWER-CALORIE RECIPES

❖ Slow-Cooker Beef Stew

Round steak or 90 percent lean beef stew cuts
1 tbsp olive oil
1 16-ounce can tomatoes
1 package frozen onions, sliced (use to your liking)
1 can beef broth
1 small package baby carrots
1 small package fresh red potatoes
1 package onion soup mix
water to cover ingredients

Sear beef in pan with olive oil, then place all ingredients in slow cooker and pour enough water to cover. Cook on 4-, 6-, or 8-hour setting.

Makes 8 servings.

❖ Sliders

1 pound lean ground beef
1 package dinner rolls
4 slices low-fat American cheese
½ cup onion, diced
Ketchup or mustard to taste

Grill 8 beef patties. Halve and toast 8 dinner rolls. Top each roll with 1 patty, 1 slice cheese, onions, and condiments.

Makes 8 servings.

❖ Sausage and Bean Soup

6 ounces turkey kielbasa sausage, sliced
1 cup diced green pepper
Cooking spray
1 can chicken broth (14.5 oz)
1 can black or kidney beans (15 oz)
½ cup salsa
Dried parsley

Sauté sausage and peppers in cooking spray over medium heat. Bring broth to a boil; add sausage and peppers. Reduce heat and add beans and salsa; simmer for 20 minutes. Garnish each serving with dried parsley.

Makes 4 servings.

❖ Slow-Cooker Salsa Chicken

4 boneless, skinless chicken breasts
1 cup salsa
1 package reduced-sodium taco seasoning
1 can reduced-fat condensed cream of mushroom soup
1 green pepper, sliced
1 red pepper, sliced

Place all ingredients in slow cooker and cook on low. Serve with 8 tortillas (4–6" each) or over 2 cups brown rice.

Makes 4 servings.

❖ Burritos to Go

8 flour tortillas (4–6" each)
1 can refried beans
½ cup shredded 2 percent cheddar cheese
1 green onion, sliced

Split ingredients among the 8 flour tortillas and roll into burritos. Store in separate containers in the refrigerator for grab, heat, and go!

Makes 4 servings.

❖ Chicken Wraps to Go

1 6-ounce package pre-cooked chicken
1 cup shredded 2 percent cheese
1 red pepper, sliced
Pinch of taco seasoning
Lettuce
Low-fat ranch for dipping
6 whole-wheat wraps

Split ingredients among the six wraps and roll up. Store in separate containers in the refrigerator for grab, heat, and go!

FROM THE 7-DAY SAMPLE MENU

BREAKFAST TO GO!

❖ Raspberry Smoothie

In a blender, mix 1 cup raspberries, 4 ounces vanilla yogurt, 1 tablespoon sugar, fiber powder (read directions on the package to determine how much to add), and ice and milk to taste.

❖ Egg Pita

Make ahead of time. Scramble 4 eggs; mix in your favorite vegetable (such as spinach) and a few tablespoons of salsa. Place into 2 whole-wheat pitas and sprinkle with shredded low-fat cheese. Heat in microwave.

Makes 2 servings.

❖ English Muffin Melt

Prepare a package of turkey bacon at the beginning of the week (you can use it for breakfast and to top salads and pasta). Toast a whole-wheat English muffin with 1 slice of low-fat American cheese. Place 2 slices of turkey bacon in the middle of the English muffin and go!

Makes 1 serving.

ON THE GO

Purchase some drinkable yogurt.

Grab a piece of fruit to go, and when you find time, sit down and savor some oatmeal.

1 lean frozen breakfast sandwich heated up on your way out the door (less than 250 calories).

Note on frozen meals: Try to consume only a few times a week.

1. Guacamole: 1 mashed avocado, 2 minced garlic cloves, chopped cilantro leaves (to your liking), and ½ chopped onion; combine ingredients. Makes 2 servings. Guacamole and hummus are great dips (in moderation). Just make sure to use something other than chips to dip!
2. Black bean dip: ¼ can black beans (drained and rinsed), chopped cilantro, diced tomatoes, 1/8 cup corn, and minced jalapeno; combine ingredients. Serve with pita chips: Spray pita with olive oil, cut into quarters, and toast.
3. Zucchini stix: 4 tablespoons dry bread crumbs, 2 tablespoons Parmesan cheese, 1 egg white, 1 teaspoon milk, 2 zucchini cut lengthwise into quarters, and ½ cup spaghetti sauce. Preheat oven to 400 degrees. Combine bread crumbs and Parmesan cheese. Combine egg white and milk in another dish. Dip each zucchini stick into liquid mixture then crumb mixture and place on baking sheet. Coat with cooking spray and bake 15 minutes. Serve with spaghetti sauce. Makes 2 servings.
4. Chocolate-covered strawberries: 1 100-calorie cup chocolate pudding and 8 large strawberries. Dip strawberries in pudding.

❖ Lettuce Wraps

2 tbsp mayonnaise
1 tsp lemon juice
½ cup seedless red grapes
Rotisserie chicken, shredded
2 large iceberg, romaine, or Boston lettuce leaves

Mix first four ingredients and place in lettuce leaf.

Makes 1 serving.

❖ Mexican Soup

¾ lb lean ground beef or ground turkey
1 can diced tomatoes and green chilies (15 oz)

1 can stewed tomatoes (16 oz)
1 package ranch dressing mix
1 package reduced-sodium taco seasoning
1 can kidney beans (15 oz)
1 can whole-kernel white corn (16 oz)
2 cups water (you can vary this for thinner or thicker soup)

In a browning pan or skillet, cook the ground beef or turkey thoroughly. While the meat is cooking, begin heating a medium-size pot of water over medium-high heat. Add diced tomatoes and green chilies, and stewed tomatoes. Once the meat is fully cooked, drain excess liquid, then add ranch and taco mix. Add meat mix to the water and tomato mixture. Add remaining ingredients and simmer 20 minutes. Add ¼ cup tortilla strips per saving.

Makes 6 servings.

❖ Soft Tacos

1 pound lean ground beef or ground turkey
1 package reduced-sodium taco seasoning
1 tomato, diced
1 cup shredded low-fat cheddar cheese
6 6" flour tortillas

Brown beef or turkey in skillet with cooking spray. Add 1–2 tbsp water and taco seasoning. Serve mixture in tortilla and top with tomatoes and cheese.

Makes 3 servings.

❖ Pork Chop Dinner

2 3–4 oz pork chops
Dry rub seasoning
1 medium bag frozen vegetables
2 tbsp olive oil
6 small red potatoes
Salt and pepper

Season pork chops with dry rub and grill. Steam frozen vegetables according to package directions; season with dry rub and 1 tbsp olive oil. Boil the red potatoes for 10 minutes or until tender, drizzle with 1 tbsp olive oil, and season with salt and pepper.

Makes 2 servings.

❖ Stuffed Green Pepper Soup

2 cans condensed tomato soup
2 cans water
1 cup green bell peppers, diced
½ cup onion, diced
2 cloves garlic, minced
1 teaspoon dried basil
½ pound ground turkey
¼ cup Worcestershire sauce (optional)
Ground cayenne pepper to taste
1 cup cooked barley

Add the soup, water, peppers, onions, garlic, and basil to a pot and heat on medium-high. In a skillet, brown the ground turkey. Pour Worcestershire sauce over turkey, sprinkle with cayenne pepper, stir to combine, and simmer until the liquid is absorbed. Add the meat and cooked barley to the pot. Bring the soup to a boil, reduce heat, and simmer for 5–8 minutes or until the vegetables are cooked through.

Makes 6 servings.

❖ Mediterranean Pita Pizza (courtesy of *Cooking Light*, with revisions)

2½ cups cubed eggplant, peeled
⅓ cup water
½ tsp dried oregano
½ tsp lemon juice

¼ tsp garlic powder
⅓ cup Italian-style tomato paste
2 8" pita rounds
3 tbsp crumbled feta cheese

Coat a large skillet with cooking spray. Add eggplant to skillet; cook eggplant over medium-high heat, stirring constantly, 2 minutes. Add water and next 3 ingredients; stir well. Cover, reduce heat, and cook 5 minutes. Uncover and cook over high heat an additional 1 minute. Add tomato paste; cook until thoroughly heated, stirring occasionally.

Place pita rounds on a baking sheet. Spread eggplant mixture evenly over pita rounds and top with cheese. Broil 2 minutes or until cheese softens.

Makes 2 servings.

❖ Sweet and Sour Shrimp Kebab

3 tbsp chili sauce
1 tbsp soy sauce
½ tsp garlic powder
8 oz pineapple chunks in juice
3 dozen medium peeled and deveined shrimp (place 6–12 shrimp aside
     for shrimp cocktail on following day)
1 green pepper, sliced to fit skewer
1 small onion, sliced to fit skewer

Combine first 4 ingredients in a mixing bowl. Add shrimp to mix and refrigerate for 30 minutes. Skewer shrimp, pineapple, green pepper, and onion and grill until shrimp turn pink.

Makes 4 servings.

❖ Grilled Cheese with Spinach and Tomatoes

2 slices whole-wheat bread
1–2 tsp olive oil
1–2 slices low-fat cheese (mozzarella works great)

2 tomato slices

⅓ cup spinach

Coat 1 side of each slice of bread with olive oil. Layer cheese, tomato, and spinach on the dry side of one slice of bread and top with the other slice. Grill in a skillet over medium heat or use a panini press.

Makes 1 serving.

❖ Raspberry Salad

2 cups spinach or favorite lettuce

¼ cup sliced almonds

¼ cup pasteurized feta cheese crumbles

¼ cup dried cranberries

1–2 tbsp light raspberry vinaigrette (Kraft makes a wonderful version of this with an olive oil base)

Makes 1 serving.

❖ Tuna Salad

1 cup spinach

1 cup romaine

1 can tuna in water

¼ cup peanuts, sliced almonds, or sunflower seeds

¼ cup dried cranberries (optional)

2 tbsp of your favorite low-fat dressing (I prefer the raspberry or balsamic vinaigrette by Kraft)

Serve with a toasted pita round.

Makes 1 serving.

❖ Meatless Chili

1 medium onion, chopped

4 cloves garlic, minced

1 tbsp olive oil
¾ cup carrots, julienned
2 tomatoes, diced
2 cans black beans, drained (15 oz)
½–1 package chili seasoning mix
1 tbsp parsley, chopped

Sauté onions and garlic in oil in a large skillet. Add remaining ingredients; cook over medium heat for 10–15 minutes. Serve with a handful of tortilla chips.

Makes 6 servings.

❖ Tex-Mex Salad (courtesy of Weight Watchers)

1 (15 oz) can no-salt-added black beans, rinsed and drained
¼ cup chopped green onions
¼ cup frozen whole-kernel corn, thawed
½ cup salsa
8 cups shredded romaine lettuce

Combine beans, green onions, corn, and salsa. Spoon bean mixture over 2 cups shredded romaine lettuce.

Makes 4 servings.

NOTES AND SOURCES

1   Lenita Anthony, *ACE's Guide to Pre-Natal Fitness* (DVD). California: Healthy Learning, 2004.

2   Lenita Anthony, *Pre- and Post-Natal Fitness: A guide for Fitness Professionals from the American Council on Exercise.* California: Healthy Learning, 2002, p. 13.

3   James F. Clapp III, *Exercising Through Your Pregnancy: Your Guide to an Active, Healthy Pregnancy.* Nebraska: Addicus Books, 2002, p.160.

4   Elizabeth M. Ward, *Expect the Best: Your Guide to Healthy Eating Before, During and After Pregnancy.* Hoboken, NJ: John Wiley & Sons, 2009, p. 114.

5   KidsHealth.org, "Preparing for Multiple Births." The Nemours Foundation, 1995–2010 (http://kidshealth.org/parent/pregnancy_newborn/pregnancy/multiple_births.html).

6   Clapp, *Exercising Through Your Pregnancy*, p. 91.

7   Ibid.

8   Anthony, *Pre- and Post-Natal Fitness*, p. 36.

9   Sara Kooperman, *Moms in Motion: Pre/Post Natal Exercise Certification* (Sarah's City Workout, 2000), p. 44.

10 Clapp, *Exercising Through Your Pregnancy*, p. 20.

11 Kooperman, *Moms in Motion*, p.35

12 Ibid., p. 12.

13 Scott Josephson, *Women Metabolism, and the Hormonal Highway* (live conference). IDEA Health & Fitness Association, 2010.

14 From various studies, mostly Clapp, Exercising Through Your Pregnancy.

15 Bonnie Fremgen, Suzanne Frucht. *Medical Terminology: A Living Language*, 4th ed. Upper Saddle River, NJ: Prentice Hall, 2008.

16 Ibid.

17 Ward, *Expect the Best*, p. 55.

18 Ibid.

19 The American Dietetic Association and Elizabeth M. Ward. Pregnancy Nutrition: Good Health for You and Your Baby. Hoboken, NJ: John Wiley & Sons, 1998.

20 Institute of Medicine, *Nutrition During Pregnancy: Part I: Weight Gain, Part II: Nutrient Supplements* (Washington, DC: National Academies, 1990).

21 The American Dietetic Association and Ward, p. 20

22 Ward, *Expect the Best*, p. 33.

23 Ibid., p. 36.

24 Ibid., p. 36

25 Ibid., p. 35

26 The American Dietetic Association and Ward, *Pregnancy Nutrition*, p. 9

27 Ibid., p. 29

28 Ward, *Expect the Best*, p. 56

29 Ibid.

30 Ibid., p. 62.

31 Ibid., p. 60.

32 Ibid., p. 39.

33 Gwen Hyatt, *Exercise and Urinary Incontinence*. Tucson, Arizona: Desert Southwest Fitness, Inc., 2003, p. 4.

34 Ibid., pp. 12, 25, 26, 36.

35 Clapp, *Exercising Through Your Pregnancy*, pp. 72, 73, 74.

36 The American Dietetic Association and Ward, *Pregnancy Nutrition*, p. 134.

37 Ward, *Expect the Best*, p. 134.

38 Ibid., p. 39.

39 Ibid., pp. 26, 28, 32–36, 41, 43, 45.

40 ACOG Committee Opinion Number 267, January 2002, reaffirmed 2009.

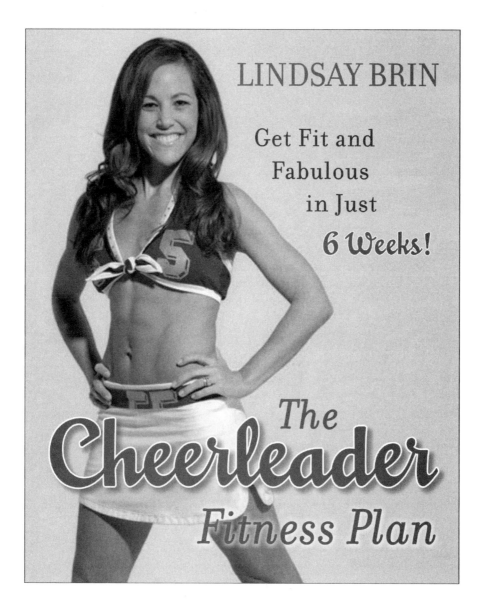
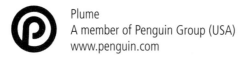